W9-CAF-979

THE 6 WEEK CURE FOR THE MIDDLE-AGED MIDDLE

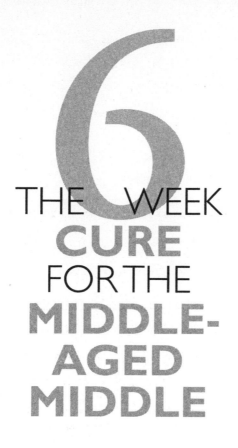

THE 6 WEEK CURE FOR THE MIDDLE-AGED MIDDLE

Mary Dan Eades, M.D., and Michael R. Eades, M.D.

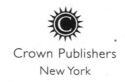

Crown Publishers
New York

Copyright © 2009 by Nutridox LLC.

All rights reserved.

Published in the United States by Crown Publishers,

an imprint of the Crown Publishing Group,

a division of Random House, Inc., New York.

www.crownpublishing.com

CROWN and the Crown colophon are registered trademarks of Random House, Inc.

Library of Congress Cataloging-in-Publication Data

Eades, Michael R.

The 6-week cure for the middle-aged middle / Michael R. Eades and Mary Dan Eades.—1st ed.

1. Reducing diets.   2. Middle-aged persons—Health and hygiene.   3. Abdomen.

I. Eades, Mary Dan.   II. Title.

RM222.2.E15 2009

613.2'5—dc22   2008048876

ISBN 978-0-307-45071-5

Printed in the United States of America

Design by Chris Welch

10 9 8 7 6 5 4 3 2 1

First Edition

We dedicate this book to our siblings,

ROSE, LARRY, DAVID, TIM, JAYNE, AND JANET,

who've been with us
throughout life's stages and roll with us
now through middle age

ACKNOWLEDGMENTS

Books are not solitary works; they come about through the efforts of not only their authors, but also an entire cast of others who contribute to the process. This book is no exception, and we would like to gratefully acknowledge the many contributions of the other people who made the idea of this book manifest.

First, as always, we thank our faithful agents, Channa Taub and Carol Mann, both for finding a great publishing home for this book, but also for their friendship, loyalty, and tireless efforts on our behalf over the last dozen years.

We appreciate all the efforts of our editor, Heather Jackson, who made this book better by her insight and liberal application of her blue pencil (though it was actually red). Kudos and gratitude to our copy editor, Carole Berglie, who caught everything that Heather's eagle eye missed and kept us honest. And thanks as well to all the folks at Crown Publishing who worked to get the manuscript beautifully between two covers and into stores everywhere.

To our long-time assistant, Kristi, we owe endless gratitude. It is she who makes sure everything else gets done when we have to focus on writing. We would never make it without you, KB. We'd never want to try!

Many thanks to our favorite graphic artist, Faith Keating, for the figures in Chapter 3.

To our readers, both of blogs and books, we tip the hat as well. Some of you have been faithfully reading what we've written since *Thin So Fast* in 1989, twenty years ago. Others came aboard with *Protein Power* in 1996, but that's now a dozen years ago as well. We treasure knowing our work has been of help to you, as evidenced by the kudos and kind words you've written to us, but even more important we appreciate that you question us and keep us striving to stay ahead of you. Most of all, we appreciate your loyalty and intelligence.

And to our family, our sons, daughters-in-law, and wonderful grandchildren, who love and support us unstintingly, and whom we love and appreciate above all things in the world. Know that everything we do, the good stuff anyway, we do for you.

CONTENTS

PART II

INTRODUCTION

B ob Hope famously quipped that middle age is when your age starts to show around your middle, and the audience always obliged him with a hearty laugh. But for millions of adults the sad irony of the middle-aged middle is anything but funny. Except for a select few metabolically gifted individuals, crossing the threshold into middle age heralds the beginning of a battle of the bulge that seemingly never ends. Granted some reach that threshold sooner than others; some acquiesce to the larger belt and the broader silhouette with some degree of aplomb, while others rail against time and fate. They take up and discard first one diet and exercise program and then the next in a frustrating quest to recapture the slender waist they can still recall, but no longer see in the mirror.

We've spent the majority of our medical careers helping people of every description with just this battle, combating overweight and weight-related health issues. Although some were in their teens and twenties, and some were in their seventies and eighties, the vast bulk of the many thousands of patients we guided to better health and lower weights were in middle age. What we learned from these many years in the diet trenches is that middle-aged weight is stubborn; it's different to deal with; it doesn't respond readily to modest dietary changes or the incremental increases in exercise usually recommended by the purveyors of received medical and nutritional wisdom. The factors driving middle-aged weight gain—which really does go straight to the middle—are like a perfect storm, metabolically speaking. A confluence of changes in hormones, stress, lack of sleep, alcohol intake, medications, fat and cholesterol phobias, and a mountain of nutritional misinformation combine to create a mid-life tsunami that seems to swamp the metabolism and fill every nook and cranny of the middle of the body with fat.

For more than twenty years we have researched this area of science, refining the tools to deal with it effectively, writing about it, and lecturing on it, so you'd think that our expertise would protect us from the tsunami, if it came our way. But it didn't. Like everyone else, when the middle-age wave hit, we found ourselves floundering in the tide, paddling as fast as we could, and still not making much headway. At least not until we dug back into the medical bag of tricks we had used with success in our middle-aged patients and applied them to ourselves. Here's how it all began.

MIKE'S STORY

Our wake-up call came the morning we walked onto the set to film the pilot for our TV cooking show. Years before, I had gained a tremendous amount of weight while pursuing my career as a busy, practicing physician, then lost it on a diet I cobbled together from information I got rereading my old medical school texts and delving into the medical literature. My weight loss did not go unnoticed by my patients, and soon many were clamoring for me to put them on the same diet I had developed for myself. I did so with great success. In short order my practice changed. My wife, Mary Dan, left her busy family practice and joined me in what became a huge bariatric (the treatment of obesity) practice. We refined the original diet and wrote about our methods in *Protein Power,* a book that sold over 4 million copies. During the never-ending promotion of the book, we met a producer who proposed that we star in a TV cooking show designed around the precepts of our diet and a cookbook we had written. We said, "Let's do it." He put the deal together and set the shooting schedule for the pilot.

We walked onto the set in sunny Southern California one morning filled with both enthusiasm and apprehension. As we wandered through the semi-organized chaos that is a film studio, stepping over giant cables, ducking under the scaffolding for the overhead cameras, and dodging production assistants darting here and there, we began to wonder what we had gotten ourselves into. The whirlwind of activity and the thirty or so people on the set were intimidating, to say the least. We had done countless live and taped television and radio interviews in the previous years, but never a project in which we were the sole actors on the stage, the ones who had to carry the entire show on our own shoulders. A young man recognized us and directed us to the Green Room, telling us the director would be in to talk with us shortly.

The director, a total stickler for every aspect of the production, didn't mince words when he joined us in the Green Room. "We're going to have to do something," he said. "You guys are too fat to be starring in this kind of a cooking show."

We were stunned. I was a much lesser version of my former fat self and thought of myself as pretty slender. Mary Dan had gained a little weight in the ten years since the publication of *Protein Power,* but certainly wouldn't have been considered fat by anyone's estimation. People we met at lectures, book signings, and other appearances uniformly commented on how thin and healthy we looked and always added that we were good advertisements for our diet.

"Yeah, well, it doesn't work that way on TV," said the producer. "If you're the stars of a show on healthy eating, you've got to be thin.

Granted, you look better than the average Joes and Janes out there, but they don't have their own health show. TV is a youth-driven medium. You've got to look young to make it on TV and young means thin, especially around the middle. It's like the golfer, Lee Trevino, says: the young guys are the 'flat bellies.' You've got to have a flat belly if you want to make it in this biz. The camera is going to put 10 pounds on you, and you've both got bellies starting out. Imagine 10 pounds added to that."

Bellies . . . ?

"When you do lectures you're dressed up, right? You wear suits, don't you?"

We nodded.

"At book signings you sit behind a desk, shake a few hands and sign books. It doesn't work that way on TV. You're going to be moving around, bending over, putting stuff in the oven; you're going to be seen from all angles. If we try to hide the fact that you've got a little extra weight around the middle, which will be hard since the camera will magnify it, the viewers will know. Putting you in baggy sweaters or loose clothing will just make them think you're fat and trying to disguise it, and the show will lose all credibility."

In a flash, Mary Dan and I had both gone from being confident in our own 50-plus-year-old bodies to being aware of the small paunches that had suddenly seemed to materialize out of nowhere. What before had seemed nothing more than a little tightening of the waistband now suddenly assumed Falstaffian proportions.

"What can we do?" we asked. "If we try to hide it, they'll think we're fat; if we don't, they'll know for sure. It's a catch-22. We can't win."

Our director said, "I haven't worked in this biz for over forty years and not learned a trick or two. Here's how we're going to make this work. Since you, Mary Dan, are going to be the main cook, we'll keep you standing behind the counter. You're short enough that with the height of the counter and a little work with wardrobe we can keep you covered without appearing to do so. Mike, we'll have you do all the moving and bending, so you're going to have to take the bullet."

"Take the bullet? What do you mean?"

He reached into his large canvas bag and pulled out what appeared to be a giant piece of black foam rubber. "Before you go to wardrobe, let me help you put this on under your tee-shirt."

The giant piece of foam rubber turned out to be a device called an abdominal censure; in other words, a giant girdle.

"I can't wear that . . ." I said.

"Hey, don't think you're the Lone Ranger," he replied. "Why do you think I have this? I didn't buy it just for you. A surprising number of the people you see on TV daily are wearing one of these. Lift up your shirt."

"Who?" I asked.

"I'm not going to tell anyone about you, and I'm not going to tell you about anyone else. Lift your shirt."

I lifted my tee-shirt; he wrapped the thing around my abdomen and put his knee in the middle of my back to cinch me in. Feeling a little like the male equivalent of Scarlett O'Hara in the corset scene, I dropped my tee-shirt down and looked in the mirror. I had to admit, I looked better.

I wore the girdle and Mary Dan stayed behind the counter for the two days it took to film the pilot. (Now we shoot two shows per day, but then we were raw beginners.) Our show got picked up by PBS and we scheduled to start shooting about three months later. Fortunately, the pilot was shown only to others in the industry, and now the show with me squeezed into neoprene and Mary Dan cloistered behind the counter has been relegated to the never-to-be-shown file. What we took away from that day was the certainty that something had to be done and quickly . . . but what?

NOT LONG AFTER returning home from this experience we attended a large charity event at which we were seated at a table with several middle-aged women. One was significantly overweight, but the others would be considered within or close to their normal weight range. The discussion turned to weight loss. The constant thread through the conversation was how much easier it was to lose weight overall, compared to the difficulty of losing it in the waist. All the women bemoaned their stubborn middles.

Meanwhile, still stinging from our recent brush with abdominal truth, we had begun looking at the midsections of nonobese middle-aged men, and it quickly became clear that they all had paunches of various sizes. It appeared that there were no (or damned few) middle-aged flat bellies out there of either gender. Young people who were a little overweight didn't seem to have protuberant guts; they carried their excess weight all over. But in middle age it went straight to the middle. Even young people with guts don't look the same as middle-aged people with big bellies; there is a difference, easily recognized. We realized that our director had been right; it's not just normal body weight, but a flat belly that is the real sign of youth, so we set out to get one. Drawing on two decades of experience in clinical practice, helping thousands of patients of all ages, we dusted off and examined every weight-loss trick in our armamentarium. We did the same thing we had done years before when we did our research for *Protein Power,* combing the worldwide medical literature for insight and scientific substance, but instead of concentrating on weight loss in general, we focused our search on abdominal weight loss—more specifically, abdominal *fat* loss. We discovered that, although spot reducing is impossible, the diameter of the midsection can be reduced quickly with the right nutritional tools. Fortunately, many of those tools dovetailed perfectly with those we'd used successfully over the years with patients in our clinical practice. After a couple of weeks of intense effort, we put together a flat-belly program for ourselves that combined a reworking of our old *Thin So Fast* and *Protein Power* diets that we had used in many thousands of patients, a number of nutritional supplements we had learned about from our wide-ranging medical research in the intervening years, and a unique, but simple, abdominal exercise plan based on the laws of physics.

We had exactly six weeks before our next shoot, so we launched into the program with full vigor, with the goals of avoiding the dreaded cinch and the safety of the counter. The regimen vastly exceeded our expectations. The greatest changes occurred in the first two weeks with smaller, but still significant, changes taking place over the course of the next four weeks. We appeared for the shoot with flat bellies, much to the delight of our director, and we were able to move from refrigerator to sink to counter, showing full physique and with nary a trace of neoprene. We no longer had to suck it in every time we changed positions for fear that the camera might catch our midsections at an unfavorable angle. The regimen had been a slam dunk.

It's been a little over two years (and twenty-six episodes of our show) since we developed and took "The 6-Week Cure" ourselves, but our success has inspired countless readers, viewers, relatives, patients, friends, and friends of friends to want to know exactly how we did it. This book provides those answers. In it, you will discover not only what happens in middle age that drives fat into your middle body, but more importantly, what you can do, physically and nutritionally, to harness the metabolic forces at work and turn the tide. With a little hard work over a very short stretch, you, too, can regain a more youthful silhouette. When you do, we're sure you'll agree with what we discovered: there's nothing that restores youth like curing your middle-aged middle.

PART

1

PROFILES IN HISTORY

*"Our brains are hardwired. The cortex in the back of our brains scans
the environment looking for fertile mates."*
—Louann Brizendine, M.D.,
author, *The Female Brain*

I f you believe the attractiveness of a slender body and especially a flat abdomen are a recent Western, industrialized-countries phenomenon, history will prove you wrong. In cultures around the world and across the millennia, a slender middle as the hallmark of health, vigor, and beauty has nearly always headed the list of desirable physical attributes in a mate.

Take, for example, Queen Hatshepsut, fifth pharaoh of the eighteenth dynasty of Egypt and the most powerful woman in her world. She died at age 50 from a ruptured tooth abscess, an ignominious end to be sure. That notwithstanding, as she was borne to her grave a hoary, desiccated corpse, swaddled in folds of her own fat, her funeral procession passed myriad statuary and glyphs representing her, not as she was but as she wished to be: young, sleek, and of slender silhouette. Modern analysis of her mummified remains, however, tells us such was not the case. Middle age had caught up to the queen. It appears that along with being quite obese, she had wretched teeth, bones riddled with tumors, and may have suffered from diabetes as well. Yet during her lifetime and for all the many centuries since her death, her svelte form in statues and paintings belied the middle-aged sprawl of the real Hatshepsut.

In 1991, feminist Naomi Wolf opined, "Beauty is a currency system like the gold standard. Like any economy, it is determined by politics, and in the modern age in the West it is the last, best belief system that keeps male dominance intact." In other words, Ms. Wolf views our opinion of beauty as being based not on any innate or inborn sense of what is attractive, but as a product of our cultural indoctrination. We think a pretty face is pretty or a flat belly is attractive for no other reason than that's the way we've been programmed to think by the society in which we live. The covers of *Playboy*, *Playgirl*, *Vogue*, and *Cosmopolitan*, she claims, set our standards for attractiveness, not the reverse. According to Wolf and others of her opinion, there is no universal standard for human beauty. Were we not programmed by advertisers and the entertainment industry, we would find a fat man or woman just as attractive and desirable as a thin one.

We disagree.

Years of serious scientific study, across numerous disciplines, prove otherwise. Our attraction to a pretty face and a flat belly is in our genes and is an atavistic throwback to a time when such features represented health and the ability to reproduce—important requirements in the selection of a mate. As Harvard Professor Deirdre Barrett puts it, these deep-seated universal standards of beauty "reflect our evolutionary need to estimate the health of others from their physical characteristics."

It's not our cultural programming that sets our standards for beauty; it is our instinct.

As recently as seventy-five years ago there were no reliable antibiotics available to fight bacterial infections and absolutely nothing to deal with myriad other infectious agents to which we humans fall prey. Many diseases common to our great-grandparents' generation and be-

fore are virtually never seen now. And many of these diseases left dis-
figuring marks on their victims. For instance, it was common in those
days to see people with terrible scarring from smallpox, along with ring-
worms and running sores from other skin infections. The peaches-and-
cream complexions of persons of the opposite sex advertised their
health. Who wouldn't be more attracted to someone with smooth, un-
blemished skin? Rickets and other diseases struck their marks on the
bones, leaving their victims with obvious physical deformities. Who in
choosing a mate wouldn't be more attracted to someone with a sym-
metrical physique and straight posture? And women who were youthful and flat of belly were more fertile and therefore more attractive as
mates. This all sounds cruel, but unfortunately biology *is* cruel. Our
ideas of beauty are not driven by Madison Avenue, but by the microchip
in our DNA, placed there by Mother Nature using her most indispensa-
ble tool: natural selection.

But is Mother Nature's handiwork accurate? Does it apply today? Or
is it an artifact of evolution like the vestigial tails on some apes? We
would argue that it is accurate. At least the part that makes us perceive
a thin waist as more desirable than a thick one.

Our hard-wiring compels us to be drawn to potential mates with
slender midsections because we are drawn to health. Although we may
not perceive it at a conscious level, at the DNA level we want to mix our
genes with those of someone who is healthy. That innate desire trans-
lates to our brains' singling out those with narrow waists and deeming
them attractive. And with good reason. As it turns out, those flat abdomens usually reside on healthy people.

For over a century scientists have known that the forces of natural selection have molded our bones, muscles, organs, biochemistry, and
physiology to provide optimal health under our evolutionary circumstances. Those who didn't adapt died off. Those who made the cut
are the ancestors of we who are alive today. About forty years ago
researchers started applying the laws of natural selection, not just to
physical adaptations, but to mental adaptations as well. Evolutionary

psychologists realized that animals born with instinctive fears—for example, fear of falling or fear of snakes or fear of the dark—had a greater likelihood of surviving and passing on those inbred fears to their progeny. In the same way, desires were genetically hardwired. Those who developed the instinct to search for mates using looks and/or body size and shape as indicators of good reproductive health were more likely to populate the world with their offspring who carried these same genes.

Dr. Donald Symons, one of the founders of evolutionary psychology, opines that "the tendencies to find healthy people and young women attractive are relatively 'innate' because they are universally associated with reproductive value." And he notes "males should be attracted most strongly by females of 23–28 years, since they are most likely to produce a viable infant." It so happens that healthy women between the ages of 23 and 28 years old have flat abdomens and waist-to-hip ratios (WHR, or the waist circumference divided by the hip circumference) of about 0.7. A survey looking back at all the Miss Americas for the past nine decades shows their waist-to-hip ratios have been pretty much the same from the 1920s to the 2000s, averaging about 0.7. Although these young women have varied in weight and height over the years, the WHR has remained constant.

But it's not just young American pageant contestants who are idealized as the paragons of youthful good looks and health. Across the world and across multiple cultures, the small waist and the low WHR are associated with beauty. (In fact, the WHRs of *Playboy* centerfolds and Miss Hong Kong have each tracked precisely in that range since 1987.) A cadre of researchers throughout the world have investigated numerous societies, contemporary and ancient, and found that a small WHR is desirable to members of the opposite sex across both time and culture. According to one of the leading investigators in the field "waist size is the only scientifically documented visible body part that conveys reliable information about reproductive age, sex hormone profile and risk for major diseases."

Some physical characteristics or manifestations of disease are pretty obvious. Take the sixteenth-century reformer and author Ulrich von Hutten's description of the signs and symptoms of syphilis, a disease called the "Great Pox" and common to his age: "Boils that stood out like Acorns, from whence issued such filthy stinking Matter, that whosoever came within the Scent, believed himself infected. The Colour of these was of a dark Green and the very Aspect as shocking as the pain itself, which yet was as if the Sick had Laid upon a fire." This gruesome picture was nature's not so subtle way of alerting the dating population that one so afflicted probably wasn't the best mate material. Other signs are not so obvious. At least not on a conscious level.

The WHR is a subtle sign consciously, maybe, but a strong sign at the subconscious or innate level. Why? Probably because there is a link forged by eons of natural selection between our subconscious sense of another's health and that person's WHR. The correlation between WHR and reproductive health and overall healthiness is so precise that even tiny variations in this measurement herald significant changes in multiple components of fitness.

For example, multiple autopsy studies on young women who died from nonnatural causes show a significant increase in latent disease when WHR increases above 0.8. The victims were unaware they were so afflicted because the disease processes weren't far enough along to cause symptoms, but they were present in the early stages. To show just how subtle this change is, a slender young woman with a 22.5-inch waist and a 32-inch hip circumference and a 0.7 WHR would have to increase her waist circumference to only 25 inches, a mere 2.5 inch increase (which represents in increase of only ¾ inch from front to back) to increase her WHR to 0.8 and increase her chances of disease.

Sex hormones drive the distribution of fat to and from various anatomical areas. Prior to puberty women have WHRs that are about the same as young males, and as they reach menopause, they once again approach the male WHR range (around 0.9). During their fertile years estrogen inhibits the deposition of fat in the abdominal area and shifts it to the hips and thighs, thus the lower WHR. And, what's more, a normal WHR is associated directly with increased fertility. Studies have shown that women with WHRs above 0.8—independent of body weight—have significantly reduced pregnancy rates than do women with WHRs in the 0.7–0.79 range.

But a lower WHR is not just a sign of fertility. As mentioned above, it is a sign of good physical health all around. And it may even be an indicator of mental health as well. Some studies have shown that higher WHRs correlate with increased vulnerability to stress and a higher prevalence anxiety and depression than normal WHRs.

Many parasitic diseases such as schistosomiasis, leishmaniasis, amoebiasis, and others cause a swelling of the abdomen without an overall weight gain. These diseases and many others are still prevalent in undeveloped countries, and would have been a common part of our evolutionary heritage. The increase in WHR occasioned by an infection or infestation with one or more of these parasites would be an indication of less than stellar health and would undoubtedly have raised a subtle cause for concern in potential mates.

In view of our modern medical evidence it seems pretty obvious that an increase in WHR—even a slight one—should give us insight into the overall health status of another, but that's today. What about in ancient times? How could early man (or woman) recognize these subtle changes as portraying a less than perfect mate, at least from a health perspective? No one knows with certainty how people in centuries past could suss out slight variations in WHR, but the evidence is pretty clear that they did. And the same goes for most non-Westernized societies today.

Dr. Devendra Singh from the University of Texas studied the WHR of members of a couple of isolated herder-gatherer tribes in southern India and found them to be in the same average range as Caucasian men and women. A number of members of one of these tribes had moved to the city to work as laborers and had been exposed to Western media. Dr. Singh queried subjects who were city dwellers and those who stayed in their remote environment about the body types each felt to be the most attractive. He did so by showing adult males from both groups photos of female nudes of varying sizes and shapes. These photos were a set that had been used by other researchers in published work evaluating the body size and shape preferences of Western males. Since Dr. Singh's Indian subjects were illiterate, he had them look at the photos and draw a line on a sheet of paper to express their opinions of the attractiveness of the women portrayed in the set of photographs—a long line for very attractive and a short line for less attractive. As Dr. Singh points out in his published research, "the results showed that the attractiveness rating was jointly determined by body mass index—BMI—and WHR. Photographs were judged to be attractive only if they were normal BMI and a low WHR." There was no difference in the judgment of what constituted attractiveness between the tribal group that had moved to the city and the tribal group that had not. Moreover, their judgments were practically identical to those of U.S. participants.

According to Dr. Singh, this is the only attractiveness study to his knowledge conducted among a tribal population using photographs of women with known BMI and WHR. Despite finding identical results between city dwellers and country dwellers from the same tribe, questions still linger as to whether or not the concept of what constitutes beauty is innate or somehow a product of modern culture. Despite their being illiterate, who knows if the tribesmen still living as hunter-gatherers have had the opportunity to be influenced by the long arm of modern media? In an effort to totally eliminate the possibility of contamination by exposure to today's ubiquitous newspapers, magazines, and TV, Dr. Singh decided to look at ancient cultures. He measured WHRs in almost 300 Greco-Roman, Indian, Egyptian, and African sculptures, and he found that across all these cultures WHR distributions varied, but the average clustered around 0.7 for women and 0.9 for men, which is the same as is regarded as ideal today.

Yet another research group took on the prodigious task of deciphering WHRs by analyzing over 300 photographs of artwork from Europe,

Africa, America, and Asia dating from the Upper Paleolithic period until 1999. As with the Singh study of statuary, this international group of experts found that the depictions of female WHR clustered in the range of 0.6 to 0.7 and have remained remarkably unchanged from 32,000 years ago until the present.

Another nascent science, or social science at least, confirms the findings of the evolutionary psychologists that a low WHR is rooted deep in our innate development as humans. Literary Darwinists apply evolution-based research to works of fiction. Since the advent of written literature (much of which, like Homer's *Iliad* and *Odyssey,* are the written version of oral literature that is centuries older), a number of themes on love, life, loss, and attraction persist with little variation across all cultures and time spans. Owing to these thematic similarities, literary Darwinists posit that these represent the inborn desires and feelings of the majority of humanity.

One such literary Darwinist, Jonathan Gottschall, from Washington and Jefferson College, writes in the *New Scientist* that folk tales from around the world contain references to females as being attractive two to six times more often as compared to their male counterparts. And a small WHR, representing youth and fertility, is a primary component of their attractiveness. Though it's likely impossible to computer-search the world's literature to determine a specific WHR from literature hundreds of years old, it is possible to look for mentions of slender or small waists. Dr. Singh's group (the same Dr. Singh who studied the statuary), along with a member of the Harvard Law School faculty, searched the Literature Online database—a database containing over 345,000 British and American works of fiction dating from the sixteenth to the eighteenth centuries—and found that when waists are described as attractive, they are described as small or narrow in 100 percent of cases. If these works of literature did describe WHRs, it is highly likely that females populating the world of literature would sport WHRs in the range of the 0.7 that we equate with youth and desirability today.

The evidence from diverse sources ranging from ancient works of statuary, to literature of the middle ages, to the research of multidisciplinary scientists tells us that throughout history, in both men and women, narrow waists and flat bellies have been deemed attractive. Evolutionary psychologists inform us that we are innately attracted to slender waists because they signal good health. The medical literature makes it clear that an optimal WHR is indeed associated with good health and that even minor increases from the optimal are associated with diminished health. A low WHR has generally been viewed as an asset of youth (although, as we will see, that constant is changing) that begins to dissipate with encroaching middle age. But why?

Why is it that as we move into our middle years our waists get larger without our seeming to do anything different to bring it about? Why can we eat anything and everything while we're teenagers and never seem to enlarge our waists, yet it appears all we have to do is look at food after we're 40, and we have to loosen the belt another notch. The next chapter will explain exactly what happens to us in middle age that increases our middles along with our health insurance premiums. And although you can't totally turn back the clock on all the ravages of aging, you'll learn that you can at least attain—and more importantly, maintain—a smaller waist and a more youthful silhouette.

2

THE EXPANDING WAIST

*"Health is beauty and the most perfect health
is the most perfect beauty."*
—William Shenstone,
British author (1714–1763)

The pundits tell us that 60 is fast becoming the new 40, that the age we consider "middle-aged" is being nudged forward by the 78 million baby boomers creeping anything but gently toward it. Younger in mind, younger at heart, younger everywhere but around our waists. There, like our grandmothers and grandfathers before us, America's boom generation has fallen victim to the curse of the middle-aged middle.

Desperate to escape the horror of a matronly or portly silhouette, we walk, we run, we swim, we march for light years on the elliptical and get nowhere. The passing years seem inexorably to pile pounds on and add inches to our bellies no matter what we try to do to forestall it. We remind ourselves that age is just a number as we pour the fat-free dressing on our meatless salads. Middle age surely won't strike us at the age it struck our parents, will it? Absolutely not, we vow! But alas . . .

What is it that thickens the waist and tightens the belt and leaves the buttons straining to close in middle age? Why do we gain in the middle at a certain age, even when we've been able to hold the line against serious weight gain previously? Why is it that even though we might maintain our high school weight, few of us maintain our high school belt size? Just exactly what happens in middle age that robs us of our erstwhile youthful form? Is it just that we eat more and exercise less as we age? Can't we simply place the blame there? To a small extent perhaps, but the expanding waistlines most of us seem to fall prey to are driven by a number of other more subtle changes taking place as we drift into our middle years.

The primary cause of the expanding middle-aged waistline is the storage of excess fat deep within the abdominal cavity, in and around the vital organs, accumulating where fat isn't really supposed to be and acting in a more sinister way than fat is supposed to act. Visceral fat is not just a passive repository of extra calories as was once believed; it's a metabolically active organ that responds to neurotransmitters and hormones and sends out chemical messages of its own to the brain and other tissues. When its accumulation reaches a critical mass, it begins to behave more like a tumor than a storage reservoir, infiltrating the organs and muscles—most importantly the liver—and, at least to some degree, wresting metabolic control from them. (Because of its importance, we devote the entire next chapter to explaining the differences between visceral fat and the relatively less harmful—though certainly not innocent—fat stored beneath the skin, subcutaneous fat.)

Of the subtle changes leading to fat accumulation in the belly, the most common is the accumulation of fat in the liver itself. If you've ever seen foie gras, you've seen duck or goose livers filled with fat. Sadly, many middle-aged human livers often don't look much different. Though it's long been understood that heavy drinking causes the accumulation of fat within the liver, it may surprise you to learn that the livers of many nondrinking, middle-aged people look about the same as the liver of the chronic drunk collapsed outside the local bar. Like those of the overfed geese, those livers are stuffed with fat. The condition has a name: nonalcoholic fatty liver disorder (NAFLD, or simply a fatty liver).

A number of researchers using ultrasound, MRI, and NMR diagnostic machines have discovered that over *one-third* of Americans— that's over 60 million people!—who have no history of significant alcohol consumption have fatty livers. When pathologists view samples of these fatty livers under the microscope, they are indistinguishable from those taken from fatty livers of long-term alcoholics. There's no difference, except by the history of known alcohol abuse—or lack thereof.

Fatty liver disorder is so widespread that it is now recognized as a burgeoning epidemic by researchers and physicians working in the field of hepatology—the study of the liver and its diseases. Although it has not become more than a blip on the tracking screens of most health writers, the media, or even many doctors outside that specialized community, trust us; it won't be flying under the radar much longer.

Fatty liver has left our shores; it's no longer just overfed, overweight, middle-aged Americans who are afflicted. Some studies report that the prevalence of NAFLD among "healthy" Japanese adults is approaching 30 percent. Most alarmingly of all, this disease process is now quite commonly seen in obese teens and adolescents as well. Almost 3 percent of normal-weight children have a fatty liver, a number that increases to over 50 percent in obese children. Among adolescents in their late teen years, the rate is about 15 percent.

The concern over this condition is driven by its potential for devastating long-term consequences. Because of the similarities between alcoholic fatty liver disease and NAFLD, we can look to the one for clues about the other, and what we see is that the damage occurs in stages. People who chronically consume too much alcohol first develop fatty livers. These fatty livers then become inflamed because fat in the wrong places is usually inflammatory. Once inflammation starts, the next step is liver fibrosis (a sort of scarring caused by the inflammation), which then, if not reversed, can lead to cirrhosis. The next step after cirrhosis is liver cancer, a virulent malignancy that has a low incidence of survival. NAFLD, it appears, may follow the same progression: infiltration of the liver cells by fat, followed by liver inflammation (called nonalcoholic steatohepatitis, or NASH), fibrosis, cirrhosis, and liver cancer.

We don't want to imply that everyone who has a fatty liver is going to end up with liver cancer—or any of the other intermediate steps, for that matter. We know that all alcoholics who develop fatty livers don't go on to develop fibrosis, cirrhosis, and liver cancer, but the odds are much, much higher than if they had never developed fatty livers in the first place. It's the same with NAFLD: just having it doesn't mean it will progress, but the odds of its doing so are significantly higher.

We know that alcohol drives fat into the livers of chronic drinkers, but what about those who don't drink or who drink sensibly? There's the rub. No one knows for sure what causes the fat accumulation in the livers of nondrinkers or modest drinkers. But scientists are starting to develop a pretty good idea.

Although there has been all the usual blather about saturated fat's being the driving force behind the problem, all the evidence points in another direction. (As we will discuss later, saturated fat has actually been shown to be *protective* against fatty liver, alcohol induced or otherwise.) Most research has shown that a couple of common components of the American diet appear to drive the storage of fat in the liver: fructose and omega-6 fats (polyunsaturated fatty acids found most abundantly in vegetable oils). The mechanism by which fructose induces fatty liver (and fatty bums and bellies, for that matter) has been pretty well worked out, so let's look at it first.

FRUCTOSE AND THE FATTY LIVER

The chief dietary villain packing the liver with fat is the simple sugar fructose, which is found in nature, but in only relatively limited amounts, in fruits and vegetables. In small amounts fructose actually has some metabolic benefit; it primes the body to more efficiently handle glucose (blood sugar). But in large amounts, fructose can cause serious problems. The natural human diet that we cut our teeth on for most of human history contained little fructose, mainly from wild fruit, and even that was only seasonally available. The only concentrated source of fructose in the primitive world was honey, which is close to a 50:50 mixture of glucose and fructose, and that source, too, was sharply limited, not to mention perilous to come by.

But that all changed a few hundred years ago when crafty humans learned how to harvest sugar from sugarcane, which gave us easy access to another naturally sweet substance that, like honey, is half fructose and half glucose. More recently, still, came the development of a method to produce sweet syrups from corn (corn syrup and high fructose corn syrup, or HFCS) cheaply and in large amounts. Like honey and sugar, HFCS is made of glucose and fructose, in combinations ranging from 40 to 90 percent fructose. The lower end of that scale finds its way into some baked goods, but by far and away the most common form of HFCS is the 55 percent fructose blend used to sweeten soft drinks and most commercially sweetened products, from pudding to baby food. The advent of a cheap corn sweetener (with a host of properties that make it more attractive than sugar to the food manufacturing world) resulted in a skyrocketing of the amount of sweeteners we Americans consume, and because the bulk of it was slightly more fructose heavy, a sharp increase in our intake of fructose in the last three or so decades.

So how much fructose do we eat?

If we follow the diet of our prehistoric ancestors—the diet on which the forces of natural selection designed us to perform optimally—we would consume at most only a few grams of fructose per day, which, apart from the occasional encounter with a wild honey cache, would have come from seasonal fruits, edible roots, and tender shoots. And those roots and shoots and fruits would have borne little resemblance to the hybridized fruits and vegetables that fill the bins in local supermarkets today, bred for size and high sugar content. They would have been smaller, much less sweet, and, of course, available for only a few months of the year. But even assuming that early humans had access to the same quality of fruits and vegetables available to us today, the fructose from these would account for only a paltry 6 or 7 grams per small apple or a mere trace from a yam versus the 22 grams found in a single 12-ounce can of soda. And that small amount of fructose from fruits or vegetables, as we mentioned, would prime our metabolic machinery to make the best use of the glucose in our blood.

But we don't follow the diet of our ancestors. In fact, we don't even come close. The single food that makes up the largest component of the average American diet isn't meat, it isn't vegetables, isn't milk, or even fruit. It is sugar and other sweeteners, primarily HFCS. According to the most recent figures from the U.S. Department of Agriculture, sugar and HFCS provide almost one-fourth of the calories of the average American diet—a whopping 150+ pounds of sugar and other sweeteners per person per year. And that amount is growing, just like our waistlines.

Sugar and HFCS make up the lion's share of this 150 pounds, which means that on average Americans consume at least 75 pounds of fructose per person per year. That converts to a little more than 93 grams of fructose per person per day—equivalent to the amount of fructose in 24 peaches, 69 apricots, or 14.5 cups of sliced carrots. That amount is about twenty times more than the few grams per day nature designed us to deal with metabolically. What's even more frightening is that because this is an average number, at least half the population is consuming more than that. The two of us—for example—eat 3 or 4 grams of fructose per day, if that, which means that somewhere in this great land, there are two other people eating 180+ grams per day to keep the average at 93.

VEGETABLE OILS AND FATTY LIVER

The case is not yet as clearly worked out for how vegetable oils* fit into the development of a fatty liver, but it's pretty clear from research on animal models of fatty liver disease that they do. We know, for instance, that omega-6 fatty acids appear in significantly higher amounts in the tissues of those study animals with NAFLD compared to their lean-livered friends. It is likewise known that omega-6 fatty acids are inflammatory, so it is not a particularly long leap of reason to assume that the deposition of greater numbers of these fats may be one of the forces behind the progression from fatty liver to NASH.

Although it's to some degree guilt by association, which makes for intriguing hypotheses to test but doesn't always prove out, it's interesting to note that the exponential rise in fatty liver disease has occurred contemporaneously with the misguided public health campaign to increase the use of "heart healthy" vegetable fats in the diet. (This campaign has been fueled primarily by the nation's being held firmly in the grip of the lipid hypothesis of heart disease, which is dubious at best. Although it's widely believed that fat in the diet leads to fat in the blood leads to heart disease, serious research—all the way back to the famous Framingham Heart Study—has failed to prove the connection, which is why it's called the lipid hypothesis and not the lipid fact. The newest research points instead to inflammation as the likely root cause underlying cardiovascular disease.) Interestingly, our overall fat intake (as a nation) hasn't changed much over the past few decades—if anything it has dropped—but the composition of the fat consumed has changed markedly. Vegetable fats have replaced the naturally saturated animal

---

* Polyunsaturated partially hydrogenated vegetable oils should not be confused with the oils from olive, avocado, and edible seeds and nuts, none of which are vegetables.

fats that had been dietary mainstays of humankind for millennia. As you'll see, reversing that trend as we do in The Cure is a part of the solution.

ANGIE'S STORY

Angie had been overweight, though not obese, since she was a teen. She was about 38 when she came into our clinic, not for weight loss but for nausea and a vague sense of fullness and discomfort in her right side. For any doctor, the red flags instantly start running up the poles when an overweight female, nearing 40, with a couple of kids, comes in complaining of nausea and right-sided upper abdominal pain. "GALL BLADDER DISEASE" is written in big letters on those flags.

We examined Angie, took a history, discovered that there was no severe cramping nature to the pain, and that it wasn't made worse by eating in general or by fatty foods in particular. Her abdomen wasn't acutely tender, but her liver did seem mildly enlarged on examination. Still, the old med school mnemonic of the four F's of gall bladder disease—female, fat, forty, and fertile—kept running in our brains and required investigation to shut it up. She hadn't eaten since the night before, so we drew some blood and arranged for her to have an ultrasound examination of her gall bladder to rule out the possibility of stones.

The ultrasound showed she didn't have stones in her gall bladder, and although her lab report showed mild elevations in two of her liver enzymes, the enzyme (alkaline phosphatase) that usually indicates gall bladder obstruction from stones or sludge was normal. The mild elevations in liver enzymes, coupled with a blood sugar on the high side of normal and elevated triglycerides—particularly with her weight—sent us thinking in another direction: fatty liver. We'd seen it many times before and knew that diet was the cause. Strangely, diet is also the cure—as long as it's the right diet.

Angie was relieved that surgery wasn't in her future and was eager to give our nutritional plan a whirl. She was delighted when we told her that diet alone would relieve her symptoms and also help her lose some weight. We started her on an earlier version of the regimen outlined in Weeks 3 and 4 of The Cure, a "nearly all meat diet" consisting of red meat, eggs, chicken, dairy, salad, and very low-starch (mainly green) vegetables. She was skeptical at first, but within a couple of weeks she returned to report that she no longer felt any nausea and had lost about 8 pounds. A recheck of her lab work verified what we knew would happen. By fighting fire with fire—or in this case, fat with fat—her liver had purged itself of the fat within its cells, and her labs had returned to normal.

THE CONSEQUENCES OF A FATTY LIVER

Whatever the cause of fatty liver—whether it's drinking too much alcohol or eating too much fructose, too much vegetable oil, too much sugar, or just plain too much—the story plays out pretty much the same way. Once the liver starts to accumulate fat, a number of things happen, all of them bad. First, a fat-filled liver can't optimally perform one of its primary jobs, which is to serve as one of the body's main centers of detoxification. In this capacity, the liver acts to break down and render harmless all manner of toxic substances, from drugs to environmental pollutants and chemicals, to natural substances such as hormones. For example, when we drink coffee, tea, and caffeinated soft drinks, it gobbles up a part of the liver's detox capacity in order to break down the caffeine these contain. If we drink alcohol or take acetaminophen, ibuprofen, or any number of other over-the-counter or prescription medications, we occupy yet more of the liver's capacity for detoxification, stressing it even further and making its job more difficult.

Even without toxic insults heaped on it, the liver has a plethora of homegrown substances to deal with. Take the hormone insulin, for instance. When everything is working as it should, the liver acts on insulin, which is a polypeptide or small protein molecule, and breaks it down into its component amino acids. The body then recycles the amino acids to make enzymes and other essential protein molecules. If the liver is otherwise occupied or the cells are choked with fat and functioning poorly, insulin isn't degraded as quickly as it should be; it hangs around in higher concentrations than normal. This single glitch in the liver's normal workings sets up a vicious cycle that leads by several avenues to fat accumulation in the abdomen and a larger waistline.

The hormone insulin is one of the body's major metabolic hormones. It is an anabolic ("beefing up," or storage) hormone designed to drive nutrients (glucose, amino acids, and fat) into the tissues. Its minute-by-minute job is to keep glucose from accumulating in the blood after meals in part by accelerating its entry into the cells to either be burned for energy or stored for later use, but chiefly by suppressing the liver's ability to make glucose. The body likes to keep blood sugar in a narrow range and releases insulin when we eat carbohydrates, either starch or sugar, in proportion to how much of these we've consumed to bring blood sugar back to normal. Eating protein also triggers an insulin release that's needed to drive the amino acids into the cells; however, protein in a meal causes a counter-balancing release of insulin's opposing hormone, glucagon, and thus the net hormonal consequence is quite different from consuming carbohydrates.

A steady diet heavy in carbohydrates (such as the USDA Food Pyramid diet, which encourages consumption of carbohydrate foods equivalent to about 2 cups of sugar a day), necessitates a high, regular insulin output to handle all that incoming glucose. This constant demand on the system eventually takes its toll and the insulin receptors become less and less responsive to insulin's signal. This dulling of the receptors is termed "insulin resistance," which mountains of medical research have implicated as the root cause of the constellation of disorders known as the metabolic syndrome, or syndrome X. Among the disorders commonly associated with this syndrome are elevated cholesterol, low HDL cholesterol, high triglycerides, high blood pressure, diabetes, reflux and severe heartburn (gastroesophogeal reflux disorder, or GERD), sleep apnea, and central obesity.

THE ROLE OF INSULIN

Elevated insulin revs up the liver's production of triglycerides, the storage form of fat. As the triglycerides accumulate, excess insulin spurs the drive to store them, especially in the middle body, including in the liver, which sets the stage for further deterioration of liver function and only makes matters worse. Under normal circumstances, calories beyond what we require for our daily energy needs should flow into storage as fat under the direction of insulin. Subsequently, insulin levels should fall as levels of its opposing hormone, glucagon, rise, signaling to the fat cell to give up its storage as we need it. But too much insulin promotes the development of insulin resistance, and the chronically high insulin level that is part and parcel of the syndrome traps fat in the fat cells by directing incoming calories onto a one-way street into storage and making it impossible to get them out. More available insulin in circulation means more fat stored inside the abdomen, which leads to some pretty dire health consequences, among them disruption of the normal levels of gender-specific reproductive hormones and cortisol. You'll learn more about both in later sections.

A large part of The Cure is designed to remove fat from the liver, allowing it to heal and perform all its tasks without compromise. The regimen eliminates fructose, which is an obvious no-brainer. And it limits—until the liver is on its way to wellness—caffeine, acetaminophen, and other substances that divert the liver from its efforts to heal itself and get rid of the fat inside its cells. Another no-brainer. But the other changes we make require a little more explanation. We want you to increase your intake of saturated fat and decrease your intake of vegetable oils containing omega-6. Here's why.

When medical researchers ply laboratory animals with alcohol, it causes them to store fat in their livers. Researchers can then treat these animals with various therapies to see what works to get rid of their liver fat. These studies are enlightening because this type of alcohol-induced fatty liver disease is indistinguishable from human NAFLD in terms of what it looks like under the microscope and how it behaves metaboli-cally. Whatever medical scientists discover that works to treat alcohol-induced liver disease should at least be considered as a possible therapy to treat NAFLD in humans.

What works like a charm? Saturated fat! When lab animals are fed saturated fat, researchers have trouble getting them to develop fatty livers even in the face of considerable alcohol intake. In many cases, ratcheting up the saturated fat intake can actually reduce the fat accu-mulation that is already there—even while the animals continue to consume alcohol.

Even more interesting than what improves fatty liver disease is what the study showed makes it worse: feeding the animals vegetable oil, high in omega-6 fats. The combination of alcohol and vegetable oil is a potent one in causing a rapid buildup of fat in the liver. But even with vegetable oil and alcohol, liver fat can be held at bay as long as the ani-mals get plenty of saturated fat as well.

But, you may say, saturated fat works in animals, but what about hu-mans? In the human world, there is a parallel of sorts in the French population, not specifically relative to fatty liver but certainly for health and weight.

The French eat a tremendous amount of saturated fat in the form of butter, cream, and tasty French cheeses, not to mention foie gras (goose or duck fatty liver) and freely imbibe good French wines, all without ap-parent untoward consequence to their weight or cardiovascular health. That finding seems so far out of step with the prevailing Western view that saturated fat is evil that the phenomenon has been dubbed the "French Paradox," as if there were something unusual about the physi-ology of the French people that protects them from the damaging effects of saturated fat intake. There isn't; their physiology and biochemistry are no different from yours. (It might surprise you to learn that there are Spanish and Cretan paradoxes as well.) But because eating saturated fat and being healthy just doesn't jibe with the expecta-tion of the fat-is-bad-and-saturated-fat-is-worse mindset, they term it a paradox. We and others like us who have witnessed first hand the salu-tary effects of eating a diet containing good-quality saturated fat don't find it a paradox at all, but rather a self-evident truth.

To further confuse the matter in the minds of the public, some stud-ies implicate saturated fat as the *cause* of fatty liver. What's going on? Is there really any evidence showing that a diet high in saturated fat works to treat NAFLD? Yes, but you don't often hear this evidence reported be-cause it goes so deeply against the prevailing grain.

To make sense of it all, you must first understand that the recom-mendation to avoid saturated fat is a knee-jerk reaction on the part of most physicians and dietitians, based on absolutely no conclusive evi-dence. Thus the medical literature is full of articles speculating on what the best diet is for reducing fat in the liver and using inappropriate studies to demonstrate the efficacy of various nutritional regimens. Not uncommonly, though, the data often don't support the conclusion. Many of these papers recommend avoiding saturated fat and eating vegetable oils instead, which is the very regimen that makes fatty livers worse in lab animals. The truth is that most of these papers are not re-ports of actual dietary studies in which human subjects with NAFLD are fed various diets to see what really works, but are a type of investi-gation called an epidemiologic or observational study, which is invalid for proving much of anything.

Epidemiologic studies are the kind in which researchers recruit a large group of people with a given disease—in this case NAFLD—and a second group of people of the same age and sex without it. The re-searchers provide the subjects with questionnaires, asking them to re-member what they ate for the previous year. Data collected in this way are suspect at best. Think about it: can you recall what you ate last week or last month, let alone last year? Yet, with this shaky data in hand the researchers then try to find differences between what those who have NAFLD and those who don't reported as having eaten. If there are dif-ferences, then the researchers report that these differences may be a cause of the development of NAFLD. For instance, if the researchers find that the group that doesn't have NAFLD reports having eaten less saturated fat than subjects in the NAFLD group, you're sure to hear the report that saturated fat may cause fatty accumulation in the liver. In reality, these kinds of studies don't prove anything at all; they merely generate ideas for hypotheses to be tested in real studies.

The only way to demonstrate the efficacy of a diet or drug is to actually administer it to people. In the case of fatty liver, the best way to determine if a particular diet works is to gather a group of subjects who have NAFLD and put them on the diet. If the amount of fat in their livers decreases, then you can say that the diet works. A couple of different groups have done this very thing and have published their results. Both groups—one at Duke University, the other at Cambridge University in the UK—found that subjects with NAFLD rapidly reduced the amount of fat in their livers on restricted-carbohydrate, high-fat, high-saturated fat diets, which confirms the findings of the animal studies we discussed previously. How rapidly did these people shed their liver fat? In the case of the Cambridge subjects (the only ones studied on almost a daily basis), they lost significant amounts of liver fat in the *first three days*.

If you are one of the third of Americans who have fatty liver—and if your belly is large and you have diabetes, glucose intolerance, elevated triglycerides, or high blood pressure, it's almost certain you do—it is imperative that you take steps to remedy the situation if a long, healthy life and a slim waistline are your goals.

In terms of enlarging abdominal girth in middle age, a fatty liver all by itself wreaks plenty of havoc. But it doesn't work alone. In the words of the late-night infomercials, "Wait, there's more!"

Along with a fatty liver, we also tend to develop an age-related glitch in gender-specific hormones and our cortisol-stress response system. What does this have to do with our middles? Plenty. An increased output of the adrenal hormone cortisol, or its release at inappropriate times, causes a loss of muscle mass in the extremities and the accumulation of even more visceral (abdominal) fat, giving us the appearance so associated with aging: a big belly and skinny arms and legs. The beach ball on stilts. Here's what's going on under the surface.

HORMONAL HAVOC HAPPENS

As men and women journey through their 30s and cross the threshold into middle age, something unseen begins to occur in many of them: hormonal imbalance. Sooner or later, the levels of the reproductive hormones, as well as important sleep hormones and growth factors, begin a slow decline.

And as if a decline in production weren't enough, as the metabolism becomes unhinged and the middle-aged liver accumulates fat, as you've learned, insulin levels rise. The excess insulin causes the liver to produce more of a substance called sex hormone–binding globulin (SHBG), which binds to estrogen, testosterone, and the other sex hormones as they course through the bloodstream. Only the free or unbound forms of sex hormones are active; the bound hormones aren't. Whenever the liver makes more SHBG, a greater percentage of the sex hormones go from the free state to the bound state and become less active. Thus, as age limits their production, elevated insulin renders what little sex hormone you do produce relatively useless.

The shift in reproductive hormone balance that begins in the 30s and peaks in the 40s and 50s drives something even more insidious: fat storage in the middle body and within the abdomen. Women under the strong influence of estrogen in their earlier years plump up to varying degrees at puberty by laying down fat preferentially below the waist in their hips and thighs. Estrogen is a fattening hormone, designed to fill up a calorie reservoir for use by a developing fetus during the childbearing years.

With age and the decline of all reproductive hormones—estrogen, progesterone, and testosterone—the target for storage mysteriously shifts and *voilà*! The middle-aged middle is born. In a fair world, the ar-

rival of that new target zone for fat storage would at least mean the si-
multaneous loss from previous stores, trimming the hips and thighs as
it builds up the middle, but unfortunately that's not usually the case.
Human biochemistry rarely obeys the rules of fair play; it just does
what nature and the prevailing hormonal signals tell it to do. The onus
falls on women to eat in such a way as to correct the signals.

Men, on the other hand, under the influence of mainly testosterone
in their early years, become leaner, building muscle and bone and shedding their baby fat as they mature into adults. Then, mysteriously when
they cross the threshold into middle age, the hormones that kept them
lean and strong wane and they, too, begin to put on middle body fat.
To make matters worse, some of what little testosterone they may still
produce, in the presence of metabolic disorders—high insulin, insulin
resistance, fatty liver, pre- or outright diabetes—which occur so commonly in middle age, will be aromatized (chemically transformed) into
estrogen. This shift further imbalances the hormonal environment,
which robs them of muscle mass, fattens their bellies and breasts, and
undermines their sexual function and libido. Correcting the imbalances helps to reset the fat storage signals to normal.

The loss of an adequate sex hormone signal in either gender changes
the body in other ways as well. Hormonal deficiency brings with it not
just a flagging libido but, among other things, an inexorable loss of
bone mass and muscle mass. It's a sad fact of aging that unless we work
to forestall it, muscle mass declines by about 1 percent per year after age
30. That means that by age 50 the average person has experienced a 20
percent decline in peak muscle mass unless he or she takes active steps
to preserve and rebuild it. Those active steps include much of what this
book is about: eating a diet higher in the building blocks of muscle,
bone, and brain and learning to exercise in such a way as to encourage
the rebuilding process. This is not so much a weight-loss book as a
body-rehabilitation plan that will trim the fat from your middle and
leave your lean body stronger. You'll learn about how to accomplish
these two goals in later chapters.

A further contributor to the hormonal havoc of both genders in middle age—at least for some people—comes from the lack of sleep occasioned by stressful years of schooling, long hours at work building a career, financial worries, and the typical sleep deprivation that's part and parcel of child rearing. Even when you think you're withstanding it, that you're "used to it," lack of sufficient good-quality, sound, restorative sleep takes a toll on body and brain and leaves a trail of hormonal disruption that we can measure in the laboratory: elevated cortisol and deficient melatonin.

TOO MUCH OF A GOOD THING

Cortisol is a hormone released by the body at times of physical or emotional stress. The hormone has myriad functions—for instance, it is the body's own natural anti-inflammatory agent. Additionally, and more important to this discussion, cortisol functions to crank up the blood-sugar production engine that turns protein into glucose (blood sugar) as emergency fuel to prepare the brain and body to meet the stressing challenge. In the absence of any stressor, the output of the hormone naturally rises and falls during the 24-hour day in a predictable pattern that we can measure easily with laboratory tests.

Quick bursts of the hormone in response to the short-lived stresses we encounter (the only kind nature really equipped us to handle) can benefit us greatly. We needed this primitive, hardwired response if required to sprint from a predator, go for days without food if game were scarce, or survive injury or infection. We need it still to leap out of the way of an oncoming truck or to react to any sudden crisis. However, what helps us in small doses now and again harms us as a steady diet. When the stress becomes chronic—as it so often does in this day and age of long hours, poor sleep, and financial, career, and family worries—this inborn protective mechanism gets stuck in the "on" position. The net result is a domino effect! The slight chronic elevation in cortisol keeps the blood sugar mildly elevated, which keeps the insulin level slightly higher, which leads to greater insulin resistance, which in turn drives the accumulation of fat in the middle of the body.

All of us aren't created equal in our ability to handle stress—at least our physiologies aren't—and interestingly, the differences seem to be tied to the breadth of our middles, even early on. Recent research has shown that among young, healthy, lean women, those with relatively larger waist to hip ratios for a given weight and height (i.e., those biggest in the middle, even when the middles aren't all that big) exhibit an exaggerated response to stress: they put out more cortisol than their slightly more pear-shaped friends.

Belly fat and liver fat wreak havoc on the stress response system, where they disrupt the hormonal balance by increasing the activity of a particular enzyme (11β-hydroxysteroid dehydrogenase, or 11βHSD) that itself acts to increase the production of cortisol, which puts the body on a metabolic merry-go-round that can be hard to stop, especially in middle age. Excess cortisol increases the storage of fat in the abdomen, which increases insulin, which increases fat in the liver, which increases belly fat, which raises cortisol—and the cycle continues. Chronic elevation of cortisol turns lean middles into fat ones at any age. So that's the explanation for the beach ball bellies, but what about the stick arms and legs?

Recall that earlier we said that cortisol acts to keep blood sugar elevated by converting protein into glucose. The body's storehouse of protein is its muscles. Chronic elevation of cortisol depletes the body's muscle mass, wasting the bulk of the arm and leg musculature, ultimately resulting in the typical aged physique: big belly, skinny arms and legs.

SLEEPLESS IN MIDDLE AGE

Whether occasioned by the demands of study, work, or new parenthood, the chronic stresses of adulthood can also lead to disturbances of our normal sleep patterns,. And lack of sleep—good sleep—brings weighty consequences. For instance, the famous Harvard Nurses' Health Study observed women over a sixteen-year span and noted that lack of sleep leads to overweight. Women who reported sleeping fewer than five hours per night were 32 percent more likely to gain more than 33 pounds over that span of years—on average about 2 pounds per year more—than those who slept longer each night.

These results surprised the researchers who began to look for explanations for the phenomenon. Their first thought was that the women sleeping less might be eating more, but when they examined that possibility, they were surprised again: the women sleeping less were also eating less . . . and yet on average gaining more weight over the years. What is this sleep loss–weight gain connection? Research suggests that it may also be a hormonal phenomenon, but in this case brought about by reduced levels of melatonin. Called the hormone of darkness, melatonin is produced by the brain during sleep in response to the cycles of light and dark that were a part of our natural human habitat for millennia—before Thomas Edison made it possible to turn night into day with the flip of a switch.

Melatonin is a mysterious and interesting hormone with dozens of actions in the body, including being a potent antioxidant that protects our brains and our DNA from attack by free radicals and our hearts from abnormal rhythms. But pertinent to this discussion, melatonin regulates the release of leptin, which is an important regulator of appetite and weight gain. Additionally, research (done in animal models of human menopause) has shown that supplementing melatonin may block the weight gain that appears in mid-life, when reproductive hormone levels dwindle. Unfortunately, mid-life is also the time that our production and release of melatonin typically begins to ebb; blood levels of melatonin in the elderly are about half those of a younger person.

That means it's even more important for those of us on the back side of the middle-aged divide to do all that we can to promote maximal output of whatever melatonin we can produce. And by and large that means lights out to get a good night's restful sleep and, if needed, even supplementing the hormone nightly to boost our levels back to normal.

The brain (actually the pineal gland within the brain) begins to produce and release melatonin along about dusk, when natural light begins to wane. The production rises throughout the evening (if it continues to darken) and peaks in the wee hours of the morning—about 2 A.M. for younger folks and about 3 A.M. for the elderly—then falls back to its baseline as the sun rises again. Light of any type, but especially blue wavelengths, will block its production. And here's where lifestyle choices come into play. What do most people do when it begins to get dark? They turn on the lights and the television and keep things all lit up through the evening, until they're ready for bed. Many people have become accustomed to falling asleep with the television on or while reading, leaving the room lit by a bedside lamp all night long. The light quite effectively blocks melatonin production, the lack of which will be a stimulator to fat storage.

Other people turn the light out and get to sleep, but often awaken in the middle of the night because of heartburn and acid reflux. They disrupt the natural dark cycle necessary for the production and release of melatonin when they turn on the light, grab the antacids, or trudge to the kitchen for a glass of water or milk. The loss of melatonin production represents a double whammy for this group of people because, not only does the hormone help to prevent mid-life weight gain, melatonin is also critical to maintaining the normal muscle tone of the lower esophageal sphincter (the LES), which is the muscular ring that tightens to keep acid in the stomach where it belongs, instead of letting it backflow up into the esophagus at night. Getting a good night's sleep is an important element of The Cure, and you simply can't achieve it if reflux is waking you up every night.

While you can't change the physiology or physiognomy you were born with, you can live your life in ways that quiet the chronic call for more cortisol and improve your body's production and release of melatonin. You can reduce the chronic stresses on your body in several ways: work to get a full night's restful sleep, turn out the lights and turn off the television before going to sleep, address acid reflux (GERD) if you have it, learn to relax during the day, and eat a diet that helps to keep cortisol levels in balance. You'll learn more about how to accomplish these goals in later chapters. You'll also find recommended resources to help you in the Appendix, including sleep hygiene tips and sources for natural GERD relief.

First-hand clinical experience (and our own individual experience as we watch that 50-year-old milestone receding ever farther in our rearview mirrors) has taught us the near futility of battling middle-aged weight gain in the face of an imbalance of hormones—particularly the reproductive hormones in women during menopause, but also the *andropause* (sometimes referred to as "male menopause") that commonly occurs in men. Although the appearance of such symptoms as weight gain, mood swings, hot flashes (power surges, we call them), anxiety, depression, sleeplessness, night sweats, body aches, brain fog, and fatigue can certainly hint at the coming menopause in women, so can mood swings, weight gain, sleep disturbances, mid-life crises, and erectile dysfunction signal probable testosterone deficiency in men. Nothing about the symptoms alone tells how much of which hormone you need to bring the system back into balance. But a good lab test can.

We like the reliability and minimal invasiveness of the saliva tests and blood spot (finger prick) tests for determining hormone levels. Without a doctor's order, you can purchase these simple to use at-home test kits online directly from the laboratory (see Resources section) for testing female and male reproductive hormones and cortisol. Many physicians maintain accounts with similar testing laboratories and may keep these same kinds of kits in their offices; if so, you could obtain them there as well. The at-home designation simply refers to where you collect the specimen, which has to be done at particular times of the day, and doing it at home or work is much more convenient that multiple trips to the lab or doctor's office. Once the specimen is collected, it is mailed directly to the laboratory, where it's tested. In most states, the lab can send the results directly to the patient; in a few, such as California, the results must be reported to a licensed health practitioner.

Needless to say, you can (and should) discuss hormonal testing with your personal physician, who may elect to use this method or may prefer another. That decision should be made jointly by you and your doctor.

A HORMONE OF A DIFFERENT STRIPE

Most everybody is familiar with thyroid hormone—or more correctly, the lack of thyroid hormone—as a cause of weight gain. Thyroid hormone, produced by the thyroid gland in response to calls from the regulating centers in the brain, functions to increase the basal metabolic rate (BMR), which is the number of calories your body uses at full rest, awake, but lying still. Thyroid hormone regulates heat production and the metabolism of food; it is also instrumental in determining how the body uses energy. Deficient thyroid hormone function can occur because of lack of production, for a variety of reasons, but one often overlooked cause is deficiency of the right kind of iodine, without which the gland cannot produce functional thyroid hormone.

It's not just the thyroid gland that depends on iodine (or its chemical cousin iodide) for normal function. Almost every cell in the body requires it in one or the other of the two forms. Unfortunately, iodine isn't particularly plentiful in the earth's crust, so there's not much in the food grown thereon. Moreover, a vast array of similar molecules in our environment competes with iodine for entry into the body, among them bromide added to bread and baked goods, fluoride now added to municipal drinking water, and perchlorate, a chlorine compound increasingly found in our water supply. To compound the problem, the iodine in iodized table salt (where the vast majority of people get most of their iodine) is only about 10 percent bioavailable and not adequate in reasonable amounts of salt to provide enough of this element so critical to normal metabolic function. The net result is that by some estimates as many as 90 percent of adult Americans may be deficient in iodine, rendering their thyroid glands relatively inactive and slowing their metabolic rates slightly. Relative iodine deficiency can be present even in the face of what appear to be "normal" readings on standard laboratory tests for thyroid hormones.

Uncovering the deficiency is done quite simply with an iodine loading test. This test, which is done at home, requires collection of a urine specimen, followed by loading with a known amount of oral iodine, in tablet form, and then the collection of all urine for the next 24 hours. If the body is replete with iodine, it will not retain much of the load; 90 percent or more will pass out in the urine. If the body lacks iodine, however, it will cling onto a greater portion of the iodine load and much less will appear in the urine. When we performed this test on ourselves— despite eating what we believed to be a diet that contained a fair amount of natural iodine from dried kelp, sea vegetables, salty foods, and iodized salt—one of us retained just 50 percent, and one 60 percent, of the iodine load. We were low; a situation we have corrected with oral iodine supplementation and switching to naturally harvested sea salt, which has substantially more iodine and iodide than iodized table salt.

Restoring iodine and iodide levels to normal is just one more piece of the puzzle that may be missing in trying to conquer the middle-aged middle. The good news is that it's an easy fix. If your doctor is unfamiliar with this test, see the Resources section for where to obtain the testing kits (which he or she can order) and reputable sources for oral iodine supplements.

RESTORING HORMONAL BALANCE

When the hormonal system is out of whack and sending strong fat-storage signals to the fat cells, losing weight effectively is nearly impossible, no matter how scrupulously you try to follow the typically pre-

scribed remedy of eating less and exercising more. If you've ever run into a brick wall in trying to lose body fat, don't feel like the Lone Ranger; in the middle years, it's more common than not to struggle to lose, despite working hard to do it. We've devoted an entire chapter later in the book to explaining why simply eating less and exercising more doesn't work and how to get substantially better results by learning to eat *right* and exercise *differently.*

Not all of our patients—in fact, not even most of our middle-aged patients—over the years have required hormonal replacement to lose fat successfully; simply following our prescribed diet did the trick. Sometimes diet alone isn't enough, which might or might not be the case with you. If hormonal imbalance is standing in your way—as proven by clinical laboratory assessment—then your first job is to work with your physician and experts in the field of "bio-identical hormone replacement" to correct those levels and get them back into an appropriate range. If your personal physician is unfamiliar with the use of bio-identical hormone replacement, you can actually find help online. We can recommend the services offered by several national compounding pharmacies, where you can consult online with experts who can then recommend a course of treatment that you can discuss with your own physician. (See Resources for online contact information.) The therapy they recommend will be tailored to your symptoms and your laboratory readings, but it will be up to your physician to actually prescribe the regimen, if he or she believes it to be appropriate to your case.

Bio-identical hormonal therapies (whether administered by mouth as pills or through the skin as a cream or gel) won't normalize the balance overnight. It may take several months of regular use (and often a little bit of tweaking of the dosages) to finally rebalance the system. The end point will be measured both by how you feel (symptom assessment by the professional) and by repeating laboratory values to ensure your numbers are in the normal range again. Then the six weeks of The Cure will give you even better results.

Granted it takes a little time, patience, and work with your health professional to get it right, but restoring hormonal balance by replacing the required amounts of the right kind of hormones can do more than relieve hot flashes and mood swings; it can restore normalcy to the shape of your body.

3

A TALE OF TWO TUBES

"One kind of obesity is restricted to the stomach, and I have never observed it in women. I call this variety of obesity GASTROPHORIA. Those attacked by it, I call GASTROPHOROUS. I belong to this category, yet, though my stomach is rather prominent, I have a round and well turned leg. My sinews are like those of an Arab horse."
—Anthelme Brillat-Savarin,
French lawyer and gourmet (1755–1825)

Brillat-Savarin, the French epicure and author of *The Physiology of Taste,* one of the world's first books on eating, had what we would today call a potbelly or a beer belly. In fact, he referred to such bellies as having among their causes the over-consumption of beer. But in his opinion it wasn't the alcohol in the beer that drove the abdominal fattening, but what he called the "fari-nacious and feculaferous matter," meaning the starchy, grain-based substances—that is, its carbohydrate content. Since Brillat-Savarin is often called the father of the low-carbohydrate diet and a great follower of what he called a reduced "farina or fecula" and sugar diet, it would make one wonder at why he, himself, had gastrophoria—a big belly. The sentences that followed the paragraph quoted at the start of this chapter begin to answer that question. Wrote Brillat-Savarin: "I always, however, looked on my stomach as a formidable enemy: I gradually subdued it, but after a long contest. I am indebted for all this to a strife of thirty years."

Fortunately, we've learned a lot of science since the eighteenth and nineteenth centuries, and even more fortunately this science can teach us how to make great strides toward getting rid of formidable bellies within just six weeks, and not the thirty years it took the French gourmet. Let's start by taking a look at the anatomical structure of a fat belly and the two types of fat that make it bulge.

MOST PEOPLE THINK that fat is fat. It's the white stuff we see around the edge of a steak and marbled into the meat; it's the cream-colored stuff that makes up the lion's share of a slice of bacon; it's the greasy yellow stuff under the skin of a chicken. We assume that our own fat looks pretty much the same and that a big, protuberant belly is made up of that fat stuffed under the skin and around our abdominal muscles. If this were true, big bellies would simply be an affront to the eyes and not to the health. But, sadly, such is not the case. Abdominal fat has a different character than that fat you might trim from a steak, which is simply storage fat. Abdominal fat is much more sinister, and even in relatively small amounts—just a little paunch, for example— gives rise to a host of problems.

When we eat too much of the wrong kinds of food and send hormonal signals to our bodies to store fat, that fat ends up in a number of places depending upon our genetics. Some of us put it on our hips, thighs, and rear ends. Others put it on the arms, upper back, and neck. Some people put it in all those places. These areas are the natural storage depots of fat, the body's closets, attic, and basement for warehousing extra stuff. As these areas fill up to their genetically predetermined limits, the body starts looking for other places to sock away excess fat, and it starts putting it in the abdominal cavity around all the organs and on a big hanging apron of tissue inside the belly called the omentum. The arms, legs, back, and neck are not particularly attractive places to display excess fat, but they are not especially dangerous places to put it. The same cannot be said for abdominal fat; it's both unattractive and dangerous.

Anatomically, the upper body is bounded by two tubes: an inner tube and an outer tube. We're all intimately familiar with the outer tube—it's called skin. And it's actually more like a plastic sack than a rigid tube, but it's a sack that holds its contents well, expanding when the contents expand and contracting when the contents get smaller. The inner tube is more like a real tube—it is the rigid muscular wall that holds all of our abdominal organs in place. It's the firm muscle we feel when we tighten our abdomens. It's the muscular wall that makes up the six-pack on the well-developed abdomens of body builders. Although we are more aware of it in the front, it completely encircles the abdominal organs and holds them in place. If it weren't for this inner tube—if all we had was our skin holding things in—the contents of our abdominal cavities would be unprotected, unsupported, and simply puddle down around our waists.

Our bodies have other tubular structures—legs and arms spring to mind. But these are different in that they aren't hollow in the same way our abdomens are. Arms and legs contain bones and muscles, wrapped in a tough, fibrous connective tissue that holds them in place much like strapping tape. Over this connective tissue–wrapped bundle is a layer of fat, covered by skin. The fat that is under the skin and outside of and around this muscular packet is called, logically enough, subcutaneous fat, or fat beneath the skin.

The fat that is between the skin covering the abdomen and the muscular wall surrounding the organs is also called subcutaneous fat because it, too, is *sub,* or under the *cutis,* the medical term for skin. Since the medical term for fat is adipose tissue, most scientific papers refer to the fat under the skin, but outside the muscular wall, as subcutaneous adipose tissue, or SAT. And since we're going to be talking about this fat a lot in this chapter, let's use this shorthand and refer to it as SAT as well just to make the terminology less cumbersome.

All humans have some degree of SAT beneath their skin most everywhere. The area under the skin is where nature wants to store excess fat. An individual's genetics determines where under the skin the excess fat will go. It seems strange that the body wouldn't simply spread the fat around everywhere equally, but it doesn't. Not in everyone, at least. There are many people with heavy arms and thin legs and just the opposite. There are people who from the waist up look normal weight and from the waist down look obese—and, again, just the opposite. It's all a function of the genetics of the individual involved. The fat distribution patterns of identical twins are remarkably, almost eerily, the same.

Likewise, it would seem that there would be an almost infinite number of places *under the skin* to put fat, and that the body would just keep stuffing it there until it could hold no more. But it doesn't work that way. Some people do indeed have large amounts of SAT all over; others don't. Whenever the SAT storehouses that the genes have provided for in an individual are full, the body starts looking for other places to cubbyhole fat. And that's when the trouble starts. That's when the excess fat starts getting poked inside the inner tube instead of under the skin, and inside the inner tube is the last place you want to be fat.

Inside the muscular wall of the abdomen reside all the internal organs called the viscera. Fat deposited inside this muscular wall, surrounding and actually *within* the organs, is called visceral fat, or visceral adipose tissue. In keeping with SAT, our shorthand designation for subcutaneous fat, let's call visceral fat VAT.

The areas where SAT resides are the normal places to store excess fat, so SAT stored there really causes no problems. VAT, however, is a different story: VAT is fat where fat is not supposed to be. And because it is fat in a place nature didn't intend fat to be stuffed, VAT acts more like a foreign substance than it does just plain old fat.

To illustrate, think of a foreign invader that we're all familiar with— a splinter—and you'll have a better picture of what happens when you start storing VAT. If you get a splinter, it gets red, swollen, and angry, which is nothing more than the visible signs of the body's trying to get rid of it. The area around the splinter becomes warm to the touch and painful—the early signs of inflammation. The white blood cells of the immune system attack the splinter, swarming around it and putting out the call for help to other such cells by secreting substances called cy-tokines. These substances function both as signaling compounds to at-tract other immune cells into the battle and as compounds that attack the splinter directly, trying to destroy it. If the splinter doesn't get re-moved, countless white cells attack it, die in the process, and produce pus. When it finally hurts so much from the pressure of the pus ex-panding around the splinter and the inflammation caused by the im-mune attack, you bolt for the tweezers (or the doctor's office) to get it removed, and in short order the problem is pretty much solved. Right after the removal the area hurts like the devil and drains pus, but by the next day it's usually almost back to normal because the mission is ac-complished: the splinter is gone. This entire train of events is the body's way of dealing with foreign substances that turn up where they're not supposed to be.

Precisely the same thing happens with VAT. Since stored fat doesn't belong in the abdomen within the confines of the inner muscular tube, the body treats it as it would a splinter. Immune cells invade the fat cells and put out the call for other immune cells. The immune cells—called macrophages—infiltrate the fat produce and secrete inflammatory cy-tokines. Unlike the splinter, which is a tiny foreign body, VAT is a mas-sive foreign body. Whereas the cytokines produced by an attack on a splinter pretty much stay within the area surrounding the splinter, be-cause it is so massive, the various cytokines secreted by the immune army attacking the VAT are of relatively enormous amounts that can spill over into the bloodstream.

When large quantities of these cytokines course through the blood they end up affecting other organs, especially the liver. These sub-stances send a message to the liver that there is a serious battle going on, and the liver responds and jumps into the fray by making and re-leasing yet another group of inflammatory substances. These sub-stances along with the cytokines from the VAT can cause a number of problems throughout the body, including damage to the blood vessels and a heightened tendency for blood clot formation. Most scientists now believe that this inflammatory process, not the cholesterol in the blood as was previously assumed, drives the development of cardiovascular disease. This explanation also nicely fits with the well-documented association of heart disease with obesity—especially of the abdominal type. But obesity isn't a prerequisite for heart disease.

In our practice we've treated many apparently slender men and women who are afflicted with the various disorders stemming from insulin resistance syndrome—elevated blood sugar, triglycerides, or cholesterol; high blood pressure; and heart disease—despite a narrow waist. Computerized X-ray scans of these patients will sometimes show that even though they have little fat in the subcutaneous layer, they have stored fat inside their abdominal cavities, albeit to a lesser degree, just as happens with the obese population. And VAT is no less dangerous to their health than for those who wear bigger belts.

The infiltration of VAT by the macrophage cells of the immune system changes the behavior of the fat itself. Instead of being fairly metabolically inert as SAT is, VAT becomes much more metabolically active. And, unfortunately, the activities it becomes involved with are not benign.

One of the more sinister things it does is to activate the enzyme 11β-hydroxysteroid dehydrogenase (11βHSD) that we mentioned in the last chapter. The 11βHSD stimulates the production of cortisol from its inactive precursor cortisone. As the amount of cortisol increases it promotes the storage of even more VAT. A consequence of accumulating VAT is that it begins to interfere with the way the body deals with blood sugar, causing glucose intolerance and even type II diabetes. It works its mischief on one level by increasing the release of fat directly into the liver (the blood vessels from the fat in the abdominal area drain into the liver), which causes the liver to develop insulin resistance, which in turn drives the liver to produce more fat itself. In a nutshell, an accumulation of VAT can lead to elevated insulin, insulin resistance, glucose intolerance, high blood pressure, elevated triglycerides (fat in the blood), and a pro-inflammatory state. It can also cause the blood to become "sticky" and more prone to clot, which is bad news for the coronary arteries.

And this bad news doesn't even include how unsightly VAT appears in the form of a giant protruding belly. Don't get us wrong. We're not saying that carrying too much SAT is all that comfortable, healthy, or attractive, either. The difference is that extra SAT padding seems a more youthful sort of overweight, whereas a potbelly screams middle age. But it doesn't mean the problem is confined to those of us in middle age.

Currently we are experiencing an explosive, global epidemic of childhood and teen obesity. There are fat kids everywhere you look, but they carry their fat differently. Just a quick glance at the silhouette of a fat teenage boy, who has his full adult height, tells you in an instant it's a teenager. If you see an overweight mother and her teenage daughter with a puff of fat spilling over the top of the girl's low-rise jeans, you can tell at a glance which is the daughter and which is the mother by profile alone. Youthful fat is mainly of the SAT variety, whereas adult fat is VAT, sometimes with a fair amount of SAT thrown in as well. Although even that distinction is vanishing, as more and more kids begin to develop the health issues we once called "disorders of middle age."

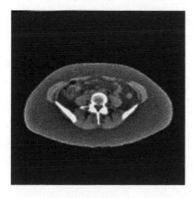 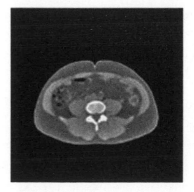

CT scan of the abdomen of a person   CT scan of the abdomen of a person
with increased SAT and little VAT   with little SAT and more VAT

Figure 1. CT Scan demonstrating SAT vs VAT

So the bad news is that when we plod into our middle years we are confronted with a fat attack inside our middles that not only pushes its way outward, giving us that large-bellied look (gastrophorous, as Brillat-Savarin called it), but is dangerous to boot. Take heart; the news isn't all bad and we'll get to the good part in a bit. Your first job, however, is to learn whether you're storing your calorie excess mainly as SAT or as VAT. But how can you tell them apart?

A CT scanner is a machine that can basically take a picture of you anywhere in your body. If you took an X-ray scan that captured a slice right through the middle of your abdominal area it might look something like Figure 1. You can see the visceral fat and the subcutaneous fat in this photo, but unless you are a radiologist, it's just a bunch of shadows. Instead, let's look at a graphic representation of the two fat compartments that will make things a little more understandable. Looking at the picture in Figure 2, you'll see the inner tube—the strong, muscular tube holding the viscera and VAT—as a heavy dark circle within the larger circle, which represents the skin. Now, let's compare two such pairs of circles: one representing a person with a large amount of VAT and the other representing a person with the exact same waist circumference, but with a large amount of SAT, it would look like Figure 3. As you can see, the people represented by these two graphics would have the same waist size, but they would have completely different fat distri-

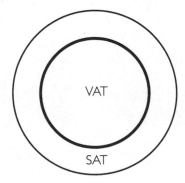

Figure 2. Representation of inner and outer tubes

butions. That's why if you simply measured the waist, you don't get the whole story, healthwise. Waist size alone can't tell you that the subject represented by Person A in Figure 3 (left) would be at much greater risk for heart disease, diabetes, and high blood pressure than the person with the same waist size but much less VAT, represented by Person B (right). But there's one more nuance here: the role of gravity.

The circles in Figure 3 represent subjects who are standing up. What would happen were they to lie on their backs? The circular representations of their abdomens would look different and more like Figure 4. Notice that the diameter of the top circles representing Person A, who has the large amount of VAT held in place by the strong muscular band, doesn't change very much when he or she lies down. A relatively small amount of SAT puddles around Person A's sides, but not enough to significantly change his or her front to back diameter. It's like a beach ball—spherical no matter how it's oriented.

Person B, on the bottom of Figure 4, with a large amount of SAT and not much VAT, looks totally different when standing or supine. Thanks to the much less rigid tube provided by the skin, Person B's SAT tends to puddle equally around the middle when standing, but falls to the sides when lying down, decreasing the front to back dimension signifi-

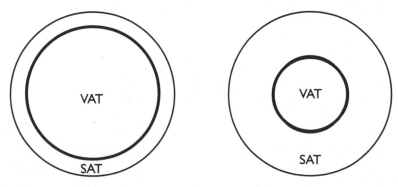

Graphic representation of increased VAT with little SAT

Graphic representation of increased SAT with little VAT

Figure 3. Comparison of large amount of VAT vs large amount of SAT

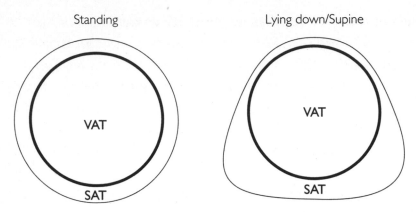

Graphic representation of increased VAT with little SAT

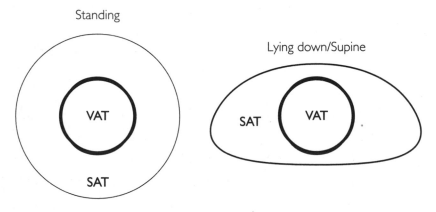

Graphic representation of increased SAT with little VAT

Figure 4.

cantly. Like a water balloon, its configuration will change depending on how it's oriented with gravity.

So, is the bulge in your middle SAT or VAT? Although an abdominal CT scan is a great way to measure the amounts of VAT and SAT, it's not a practical solution. You can't just walk into a hospital radiology suite and have yourself scanned; even if you could, it would be pretty costly.

Fortunately, there is an easier way that you can do yourself at home by comparing your abdominal diameter standing to your diameter when lying down.* Stand against a wall and measure yourself back to front, then lie down and do it again. Unless you're very thin in the middle, which is not very common in people in middle age, if you find that your diameter lying doesn't change a lot from your number standing, then you're more than likely toting a fair amount of VAT, which as you've learned can be bad news. On the other hand, if there's a spread between the two numbers, that's good news, since it means that less of your middle-aged bulge is VAT. But even if your middle is mostly VAT, there's still good news in your future.

Despite the number of serious health problems it has the potential for causing, the VAT cloud does have a silver lining. VAT is much, much easier to lose than is SAT. That's why the 6-Week Cure works in only six weeks. VAT is fat in the wrong place. The body doesn't want it there, and it wants to get rid of it just as much as you do. Given the correct set of dietary conditions the body becomes a formidable ally in ridding your middle of VAT. The body wants to store fat under the skin, which is the first place it puts it, stuffing it inside the abdominal area only as a last resort. Consequently, when you feed your body correctly and reset your metabolic hormonal balance, it will dump VAT in a hurry. And as you dump your VAT, the diameter of your inner muscular tube will become smaller quickly, reducing your waist size along with it. It is truly amazing how rapidly waist circumference diminishes once the body goes to work shedding VAT. As you lose your VAT, your SAT will tag along for the ride. In the first few weeks, you will lose some SAT as well, but nothing compared to the amount of VAT you'll lose. But if you've got some extra SAT in storage, don't despair: once you've rid your inner abdominal area of VAT and gotten rid of the fat in your liver, the SAT will start to melt away, too.

Unlike Brillat-Savarin, who subdued his stomach only after "a strife of thirty years," you should lose the majority of yours within only a few weeks.

---

* You'll find more specific instructions in Chapter 5 on how to take this measurement and a table on page 286 to help assess its meaning.

4

NOT SO ELEMENTARY, WATSON

*"The definition of insanity is doing the same thing year after year and
expecting a different result."*
—variously attributed

P ick up any magazine, tune in to the health segment of any
morning television program, ask most any health writer, dieti-
tian, nutritionist, fitness trainer, or your own family doctor
this question: How can I lose this gut? Odds are, you'll hear this advice:
eat less and exercise more. We call it the ELEM regimen, and we think
it's a fool's errand that leaves people frustrated and just as fat as when
they started. ELEM is an absolutely worthless strategy for a whole host of
sound scientific reasons that we'll get into in greater detail in the course
of this chapter. But apart from science, we know it to be a dismal failure
from our own experience, both with our patients and in ourselves.

MD'S STORY

Over the last decade, all across America, the first wave of baby boomers
began to hit their 50s. Five years ago, it happened to me. Like many

people, through my 30s and 40s, I'd fought off a few pounds here and there, but I never had what I would term a serious struggle with my weight. Twenty plus years ago, Mike and I began living a lower carb lifestyle—albeit with plenty of dietary vacations thrown into the mix— and that had always been enough restraint to keep my weight relatively stable and me in pretty good shape.

Then something happened. Despite eating the way I'd always eaten, getting roughly the same amount of physical activity that I'd been accustomed to, at age 50, I began to put on more pounds, particularly around the middle. The accumulation began gradually. When I noticed that my waistband felt tighter, I would buckle down on my diet—really watch the carbs, eschew even the occasional breads and desserts. In a week or so, I'd knock off a couple of pounds, just as I'd always done. That strategy slowed but didn't stop the upward creep of my weight and waist circumference. And this was a fresh horror for me; a thick waist is something I had never experienced in all my life. I had always been a person with a wasp waist; any pounds that had previously accumulated on me always seemed to further maximize my gluteus. No worries, I said to myself. You are a physician, with long years of clinical expertise in weight management. Just look upon yourself as you would any other patient and treat yourself accordingly. But it wasn't so straightforward.

In near desperation, I went back to the basics, turning to the famous energy balance equation, which states that change in weight equals "calories in" minus "calories out." I had already cut my "calories in" by going back to a sound low-carb diet. I assumed that I just needed to worry more than I'd been doing about the "calories out" side of things and all would be well. So I undertook a program of walking.

At least six days a week, I walked briskly for one hour, no matter where I was. At our home on Lake Tahoe, I would walk on trails around Spooner Lake or paths along the shore of Tahoe. Or I'd pedal-paddle a kayak with my legs across the water for an hour. In Santa Barbara, where we live part of the year, I would drive to a nearby beach and walk barefoot in the surf for an hour, covering about 3½ miles. At our son's house in Dallas, I'd walk the streets of his neighborhood for an hour. On the road, I'd walk for an hour at a 4 mph pace on a treadmill in the hotel gym. I did this for ten months and logged over 850 miles. And not only did I not budge the needle on the scale, I didn't lose a centimeter off my hips or my waist in ten months of near daily exercise! If I had had a patient come to my office and tell me that she had walked over 850 miles the previous year and hadn't lost an ounce, I would have been inclined not to believe her. Until it happened to me. Something was horribly wrong. I'd cut "calories in"! I raised "calories out"! Where, I asked, was the weight loss that the equation predicted?

A part of the answer can be found in the unfortunate fact that with middle age comes a disruption of reproductive hormone balance, as you learned in Chapter 2, including falling estrogen and progesterone levels in women, falling testosterone and progesterone levels in men, and the sluggish thyroid function, sleep deprivation, and rising cortisol levels that may occur in all of us. Taking steps to identify and correct these imbalances can be key to successfully whittling away the middle-aged middle. As I discovered, failure to do so can make middle-body fat loss, even on an excellent program, next to impossible. Had I not recognized this truth—that hormonal signals influence fat stores more than exercise or calories—and rehabbed my hormonal balance, I fear I would have been the one sporting the neoprene cinch at the filming of our pilot. No amount of counter or wardrobe camouflage would have hidden the camera-magnified bulge in my middle, and even The Cure might not have worked its six-week magic to flatten my belly in time to film the show.

For many if not most of you, (simply buckling down and following The Cure just as it's written will quickly restore you to the trimmer self you used to see in the mirror.) However, there will be some of you who, like me, will struggle until you take that added step of getting your hormone levels checked to determine what you need to do to get them back into balance. Another part of the answer, however, involves an inherent flaw in how most people interpret the energy balance equation. We'll examine that flaw in greater detail shortly. But first, let's take a look at why simply eating less and exercising more hasn't proved to be a panacea for obesity.

WHAT'S WRONG WITH THE ELEM STRATEGY?

Actually, nothing, in theory. The reality, however, is that it's hard to achieve, at least for most people over the long haul, for two specific reasons. The first and most important reason is that the energy balance equation

$$\Delta \text{Weight} = \text{calories in} - \text{calories out}$$

treats "calories in" and "calories out" as independent variables, when in fact they're quite dependent upon each other. We'll get into more detail about why that fallacy undermines the ELEM strategy in just a bit, but first let's discuss the other major reason ELEM fails us: hunger.

Cutting calories, the way it's usually recommended by the pillars of received medical wisdom, means a low-calorie, low-fat, minimal-protein, carbohydrate-rich diet. That structure doesn't work for the long haul because it sends all the wrong metabolic signals to the appetite control center in the brain and people just get hungry. Battling constant hunger is like hanging onto the edge of a cliff by your fingertips; sooner or later gravity is going to prevail and you are going to fall. Hunger is a deep-seated, atavistic, complex, physiological-psychological drive for self-preservation, extremely difficult to resist for the long term. In an ongoing struggle that pits human will against gnawing hunger, ultimately hunger wins. Especially in our food-driven society with a fast-food restaurant on every corner. A minority of people can prevail over hunger and lose a significant amount of weight by counting calories, but not many. And not forever.

The key in lowering calories to achieve lasting weight loss lies more in the quality of those calories than in their absolute number. The right food choices, in metabolic sync with your underlying biochemistry, can make an enormous difference between your being able to pretty painlessly reduce the "calories in" side of that energy equation or being constantly bedeviled by thoughts of food and hunger pangs. (In The Cure, we take advantage of that biochemical reality to structure a diet that satisfies appetite, maintains hormonal neutrality with regard to fat storage, and keeps hunger at bay even during a modest caloric deficit.)

Exercise, again as it's usually recommended, further compounds the problem. Few people realize how much exercise is required to lose weight. The average 150-pound, not-particularly-overweight person's body carries enough fat to provide the energy required to walk from New York to Miami without eating and still have fat left over. If this is the case—and it is—does it seem reasonable to think that you could lose much weight by taking a brisk walk for a half hour or so daily and eating even a reduced-calorie diet? Yet, that's the U.S. government's remedy for the obese of the land: just move a little more. Exercise modestly for 30 minutes a day and eat a bite less of your low-fat diet and that will solve the problem. But as I along with countless others have discovered, it simply doesn't work that way.

To lose weight by exercise requires a serious amount of it. How serious? Walking or running many miles per day, day after day. And—and this is a really big *and*—doing so *without increasing your food intake*. The big *and* is the fallacy of the energy balance equation we alluded to earlier, the phenomenon of adaptive thermogenesis, and here's how it works.

Just about everyone (ourselves included) who cranks up the exercise engine also unconsciously cranks up food intake to go along with it. It's what used to be called "working up an appetite." Most people do not realize how few calories moderate exercise burns above the calories spent just sitting around and how little food it takes to completely offset those lost calories. Walk for an hour and you will indeed burn some calories—about 180 over what you would burn just sitting at your desk. Just an extra couple of slices of cheese, a handful of nuts, or a pat or two of butter puts them right back where you don't want them, when the metabolic signals say "store." It takes a tremendous amount of conscious restraint and portion discipline not to ease those few replacement calories back into your diet. That's as true today as it was in nineteenth-century London, as William Banting (the corpulent undertaker who published a famous treatise on weight loss) discovered:

> I consulted an eminent surgeon . . . who recommended increased bodily exertion before my ordinary daily labours began, and thought rowing an excellent plan. I had the command of a good, heavy, safe boat, lived near the river, and adopted it for a couple of hours early in the morning. It is true I gained muscular vigor, but with it a prodigious appetite, which I was compelled to indulge, and consequently increased my weight, until my kind old friend advised me to forsake the exercise.

The body strives for balance in how it handles the day-to-day variations in food supply. It's a marvelous machine that can dial up or dial down its calorie burning, so as to carefully husband available fuel in lean times and waste excess fuel as heat in times of plenty. When we follow the "eat less" dictum and the number (and most particularly the quality) of calories coming in falls, our Stone Age hardwiring reads that signal as food scarcity of indeterminate duration and in short order marshals the metabolism to adjust to accommodate to the shortage. When this happens, the body cranks back its energy use; we fidget less, we unconsciously develop an economy of motion in our daily tasks, we sleep a bit more, move less in sleep, and often we perceive a drop in our sense of vitality. The body also dials back its heat production to save energy—just like turning down the home thermostat to cut the heating bill—and we feel colder. If you've ever followed a reduced-calorie—particularly a reduced-fat—eating plan, you've probably experienced that feeling of being cold. The metabolic engine slows a bit, and pretty soon the body resets its output to achieve balance with your "eating less" caloric intake. So what must happen, according to conventional dietary wisdom? ELEM. More correctly, EELEEM. You must eat *even* less and exercise *even* more. Unfortunately, if you do, your body will re-spond just as it did before, further ratcheting down the thermostat, fur-ther reducing nonessential activities such as fidgeting to accommodate. As the quote at the beginning of this chapter points out, doing the same thing over and over again and expecting a different result is the defini-tion of insanity. So what's a body to do instead?

→ EAT RIGHT, EXERCISE DIFFERENTLY

Eating right, in our opinon, most assuredly doesn't mean what it does to virtually all those health columnists and talking heads on television. In their vision, eating right means a low-fat, low-calorie diet of a little baked fish and skinless chicken and lots of fat-free, whole-grain breads and pasta dishes and breakfast cereals served with nonfat milk or nondairy soy, along with four to six servings of fresh fruits and vegeta-bles a day. That sounds so perfectly innocuous, so positively healthful, because we've all been brainwashed by that drumbeat. Now, there's nothing wrong with fresh fruits and vegetables, at least not reasonable servings of the low-sugar and low-starch ones, and certainly nothing wrong with fish and chicken, but those six to eleven servings of "healthy" whole-grain rolls and ravioli have a tremendous metabolic consequence that outweighs their caloric input: they send insulin up, which sends blood sugar down, which drives hunger.

Granted, whole grains send insulin and glucose up a little less than similar dishes made with refined white flour, but it's still a big surge upward. And upward is bad. When insulin is up, you store calories as fat and can't access your fat stores for fuel. People with insulin resist-ance and metabolic syndrome, who have chronically high insulin lev-els, will sometimes pack incoming calories into storage to a degree that leaves them without enough available calories for burning to meet the body's energy needs. (This phenomenon has been termed malnutrition or starvation in the face of plenty—i.e., there's plenty of energy in the account; you just don't have the password to access it.) To make matters worse, (when insulin surges, blood sugar falls precipitously and that's one of the strongest feeding signals to the brain, so you get hungry. That's an essential truth of human biochemistry and there's no escaping it.)

That "recommended healthy diet" has another problem as it's usually prescribed: (there's not enough good fat and protein to signal to the body that it's been properly fed, so it wants more.) The "more" available to it on most dietary regimens is more low-fat or fat-free carbs. If you give it more of that sort of fare, your insulin goes up and the diet goes bust. And worst of all, in short order you'll be hungry again. If you deny the body's request for more, you feel deprived and tired. Either way, you're hungry. It's a catch-22.

Learning to eat right does not mean denial (at least not for the long haul) but rather, making food choices that send the right metabolic signals. What you eat should tell your brain and your cells that you've been nourished, that you've had plenty. The main keys to doing that are sufficient amounts of good-quality protein and fat in a meal. Further, the calories you select should keep your blood sugar stable, should give you plenty of nutritional bang for the caloric buck, and should provide all the raw materials your body needs to do its day-to-day and minute-to-minute work without throwing the body's calorie-storage switch. By and large, that means focusing the grams of carbohydrate you eat where they'll do the least harm and the most good: reasonable servings of the aforementioned low-sugar fruits and vegetables, not in concentrated sources of starch or sugar, such as big servings of breads, potatoes, pasta, rice, oats, and sugary pastries and desserts, whole grain or otherwise.

Food isn't just calories. Every bite you eat or sip you take has an inescapable metabolic consequence. (Understanding the metabolic impact of the food you eat gives you the power to choose what that consequence will be.) In general, the protein in foods (found richly in meat, fish, poultry, eggs, nuts, and dairy products) sends a balanced metabolic signal with regard to calorie storage as well as a strong signal to quiet hunger.

The carbohydrate in food (the starches and sugars, found richly in potatoes and such cereal grains as wheat, rice, and corn, and all the things made from their meals and flours) runs insulin up, which puts the brakes on fat burning, tells the body to store fat instead, and thereby prevents successful fat loss. Good-quality fats and oils (such as the fat found in natural meats, fish, and poultry, butter, coconut oil, lard, olive oil, avocado, and nut oils) sate the appetite and provide metabolically neutral fuel for energy production.

None of this is news; we've written extensively about it over the last twenty years in our books and in our blogs (see Resources), but we were not (nor was Dr. Atkins) the first doctors in America to make the connection between eating too much starch and gaining weight. There were pioneers who traveled this road before us, some of them well known, such as William Banting, the corpulent London undertaker mentioned previously who in the nineteenth century followed a saccharine-free (meaning sugar and starch-free) diet on the advice of his physician, lost weight painlessly, and wrote the first published diet book about it. Or Vilhalmur Stefanson, the most famous explorer of the early twentieth century, who as a cure for modern ills advocated returning to the diet of the Inuit among whom he had lived for a decade while mapping the Arctic. But there were also less celebrated ones whose work you may not be familiar with. We'd like to introduce you to two of them and what they found.

THE HISTORY AND SCIENCE
BEHIND THE PROGRAM

A couple of generations ago two physicians—one on the East Coast, one on the West—while working long hours with many patients, serendipitously stumbled onto a method to rapidly decrease fat around the middle. We're sure that other doctors figured out the same thing, but these two were locally famous and published their methods. Interestingly, neither was looking to help patients lose weight.

Blake Donaldson, M.D., who practiced in Manhattan, was looking for a treatment for allergies; Walter Voegtlin, M.D., a Seattle gastroenterologist, was trying to figure out a better method for treating his patients with Crohn's disease and ulcerative colitis. Dr. Donaldson got his inspiration from a meeting he had with the aforementioned Vilhalmur Stefansson; Dr. Voegtlin came up with the same idea based on his knowledge of comparative anatomy. Though they came at two different questions from very different angles, they arrived at the same dietary answer. Both solved the problems they were seeking to solve and, coincidentally, noticed that their overweight patients lost a tremendous amount of fat from their abdominal areas while undergoing the treatment. As happened later with us and with Dr. Atkins, word of their success in combating obesity spread rapidly, and before long both physicians were deluged with overweight patients seeking treatment, completely changing the character of their medical practices. In retirement, both wrote books about their methods. Donaldson's was published in 1961; Voegtlin's in 1972. And as far as we can tell, although their years of practice overlapped, they never knew one another.

What was their secret? What did these two men independently discover? What kind of nutritional regimen did they use to bring about such great results in their patients?

Both had their patients follow an all-meat diet.

An all-meat diet?

Yes, an all-meat diet. Remember that when these physicians were in practice there hadn't been all the negative publicity about saturated fat and red meat that there has been in recent years. At that time most people considered meat as simply another food, just like potatoes, bread, or anything else. No one worried about eating it. The (misguided) hypothesis that fat in the diet causes heart disease hadn't reared its ugly head, so telling people at that time to go on an all-meat diet didn't provoke the same sort of knee-jerk emotions that it does—at least in some quarters—now.

(The patients who followed these all-meat diets rapidly lost weight from their midsections and improved their blood sugar and blood pressure problems if they had them. Calculations of cholesterol in all its various permutations was still decades away, but both doctors even used the all-meat diet for their patients with heart disease without problem. (The all-meat diet proved to be a safe, filling, rapid way to help patients lose abdominal fat while improving their health. And remember, one of these diets was developed to treat GI problems, the other to treat allergies. The rapid weight loss that followed was a surprising, but welcome side effect.

We recognize that in today's climate of saturated-fat phobia, many people will be skeptical of following an all-meat diet despite the enormous amount of research showing there is no cause for concern. To overcome our patients' reluctance and yet preserve the biochemical benefits of the all-meat diet we knew would be effective in ridding them of their middle-aged middles, we deconstructed the meat into its basic components and reassembled them in a different, not-all-meat fashion. We've modified their all-meat diet to include a selection of fruits and vegetables, carefully chosen for their minimal carbohydrate content, but micronutrient density. Using a combination of readily available protein powders and fortifying them with specific types of fats and amino acids found richly in meat, we even created a "no meat" alternative meal. We call our version a varied, nearly-all-meat diet.

Why does an all-meat diet work so well? As Dr. Donaldson explained it to his patients: "During the millions of years that our ancestors lived by hunting, every weakling who could not maintain perfect health on fresh fat meat and water was bred out." Dr. Donaldson, if his writings are any indication, was a blunt man of few words, who apparently brooked no argument from his patients about what was best for them. He's essentially correct, of course, but times have changed and we, like you, might appreciate a little fuller explanation.

(Meat contains all of the essential amino acids in the correct proportion for optimal lean tissue repair and replacement, and it has a large dose of an extremely important amino acid that accelerates weight loss.)

This particular amino acid—leucine—is in the branched-chain amino acid family and appears almost exclusively in foods of animal origin. The high doses of leucine that people get with an all-meat diet are the primary driving force behind the rapid, middle-body weight loss such diets bring about.

Another component of the all-meat diet that quickly reduces fat buildup in the liver is saturated fat. You read correctly: saturated fat. Saturated fat helps the liver mobilize and burn the fat that has collected there. As we discussed earlier, even livers filled with fat and damaged by alcohol improve with an increased intake of saturated fat—even in the face of continued abuse. Its heinous reputation notwithstanding, saturated fat is good eats, good tasting, and good for you.

If you're still somewhat phobic about eating saturated fat—and with the constant bang, bang, bang on that drum, it's hard not to be—relax. You may be surprised to learn that stearic acid, the most abundant saturated fat in red meat, actually reduces cholesterol levels in the blood. You'll learn more about its benefits in a later section. Equally surprising to you may be the new research that shows that the fat marbling in beef, far from being bad for you, is mainly oleic acid—the same fatty acid that is prevalent in olive oil and that gives it its purported healthful virtues. Even the most anti–saturated fat zealots admit that saturated fat isn't a problem when sugars and starches are limited in the diet, which they are on The Cure. Moreover, in this case, it's not just that saturated fat is not harmful, it's actively helpful in mobilizing VAT from within your abdomen.

Besides, this six-week regimen is not something you will have to stick with forever; it's nothing but a therapeutic nutritional tool, based in human biochemistry, designed to achieve maximal healthy weight loss in the least time of any program out there. It's also probably one of the easiest to follow and to adapt to normal everyday living.

If you still have some questions and want to learn more about the medical and scientific rationale for the basic nutritional infrastructure that underpins The Cure, we've written extensively about these topics in our previous books: *Protein Power* (Bantam, 1996) and *The Protein Power LifePlan* (Warner, 2000.) We encourage you to go to these sources and our blogs (see Resources) to learn more. What we'd like to do in the space we have here, rather, is to undertake a discussion of specific foods that science has shown can benefit or hinder middle-body fat loss, which is our common goal.

FOODS THAT HELP WHITTLE THE MIDDLE

While boosting protein intake in general can be helpful to sating appetite and preserving the lean body mass, one group of amino acids—called the branched-chain amino acids, or BCAAs—deserves special mention. Generally speaking, amino acids are the building blocks of all proteins. As our alphabet of twenty-six letters can be put together in near endless combinations to make all the words of the English language, so the twenty amino acids can be assembled in various patterns to create every protein in the body. Of these twenty "letters," nine (in adults) are considered essential to our survival, meaning that we cannot make them out of anything else—we must obtain them from the foods we eat. The BCAAs—valine, leucine, and isoleucine by name—are among these nine.

The body uses amino acids to construct the proteins that make up our hair, skin, nails, bones, teeth, blood, vital organs, and even our genetic code, but also, and perhaps even more important, the body assembles amino acids into the thousands of enzymes and neurotransmitters that we must constantly produce to survive and thrive. Enzymes are the critical helpers that speed up each of the millions of ongoing chemical reactions necessary for the digestion of food, energy production, glandular function, nerve signal transmission, blood sugar control, muscle movement, and on and on. Neurotransmitters are the signaling chemicals through which the brain and various tissues of the body communicate with one another, controlling everything from temperature regulation to our ability to perceive the scent of a rose.

Medical research has shown that supplementing the diet with BCAAs—in particular, the amino acid leucine—helps to prevent or slow the loss of lean body mass that often occurs with rapid weight loss, the net result of which is a preferential loss of fat when dieting. Moreover, studies show that supplementing the diet with leucine contributes to building muscle in both the under-30 crowd and those of us on the other side of the middle-aged divide. Interestingly, the addition of some carbohydrate (starch or sugar) to the diet of the younger folks actually augmented the muscle-building effect of leucine. However—and this is of utmost importance to the over-40 crowd—in older people, the presence of significant carbohydrate in the diet undermined leucine's muscle-building benefit. Additionally, recent research has shown that women, particularly those over 50, utilize the protein in their diets less successfully in muscle building than men do. What that means is that women approaching 50 need more protein for their size than men to preserve and build their lean bodies, and most of them get far less than they need. Sculpting a lean, strong body in middle age and beyond is a cornerstone of keeping the middle-aged middle at bay for the long haul. So ladies, eat your protein!

We've incorporated both supplemental BCAAs and rich dietary sources of leucine, such as whey, beef, salmon, poultry, eggs, and nuts, into our nutritional recommendations for The Cure. Aiming for an intake of at least 8 to 12 grams of leucine per day in the diet can boost the loss of middle-body fat stores and preserve lean body tissues. By taking advantage of this recent research, you'll be able to trim the fat from your middle without sacrificing your lean mass to do it.

THE TRUTH ABOUT FATS:
SOME ARE MORE EQUAL THAN OTHERS

In the not-so-distant past, the medical establishment considered all fats equally loathsome: all fats were created equal and they're all bad for you. Things have changed in that quarter, if only slightly. You have no doubt heard the drumbeat of current medical thinking on fats: some fats are now good for you—olive oil and canola oil*—but others are bad for you—trans fats and all saturated fats. That's an improvement from the old cry, but far from the truth. It seems that no matter how the story spins from the denizens of the anti-fat camp, one piece of their advice remains staunchly constant: "You should sharply limit your intake of saturated fats." The next admonition will invariably be, "which have been proven to raise cholesterol and cause heart disease." Their over-arching belief is that saturated fat is bad, bad, bad. To that, we say "baloney, baloney, baloney!"

You see with just a glance at the suggested meal plans in Part II that we've included fatty cuts of meat, chicken with the skin, bacon, eggs, butter, coconut oil, organic lard, and heavy cream in the plan. Aren't we worried that these foods will increase your risk of heart disease and raise your cholesterol? In a word, nope. In fact, we encourage you to make these important fats a regular part of your healthy diet. Why? Be-cause humans need them and here's just a few examples of why.

- *Improved liver health.* Adding saturated fat to the diet has been shown in medical research to encourage the liver cells to dump their fat content. As you learned in an earlier chapter, clearing fat from the liver is the critical first step to calling a halt to middle-body fat stor-age. Additionally, saturated fat has been shown to protect the liver from the toxic insults of alcohol and medications, including aceta-minophen and other drugs commonly used for pain and arthritis, such as nonsteroidal anti-inflammatory drugs or NSAIDs, and even to reverse the damage once it has occurred. Since the liver is the

---

* We advocate the use of olive oil, but recommend against the use of canola oil, despite its widely perceived healthful reputation. In order to be fit for human consumption, rapeseed oil (which is canola oil) requires significant processing to remove its objectionable taste and smell. Processing damages the oil, creating trans fats. Also, the oil is sensitive to heat, so if used at all it should never be used to fry foods.

lynchpin of a healthy metabolism, anything that is good for the liver is good for getting rid of fat in the middle. Polyunsaturated vegetable fats do not offer this protection.

- *Improved cardiovascular risk factors.* Though you may not have heard of it on the front pages of your local newspaper, online news source, or local television or radio news program, saturated fat plays a couple of key roles in cardiovascular health. The addition of saturated fat to the diet reduces the levels of a substance called lipoprotein (a)—pronounced "lipoprotein little a" and abbreviated Lp(a)—that correlates strongly with risk for heart disease. Currently there are no medications to lower this substance and the only dietary means of lowering Lp(a) is eating saturated fat. Bet you didn't hear that on the nightly news. Moreover, eating saturated (and other) fats also raises the level of HDL, the so-called good cholesterol. Lastly, research has shown that when women diet, those eating the greatest percentage of the total fat in their diets as saturated fat lose the most weight.

- *Strong bones.* In middle age, as bone mass begins to decline, an important goal (particularly for women) is to build strong bones. You can't turn on the television without being told you need calcium for your bones, but do you recall ever hearing that saturated fat is required for calcium to be effectively incorporated into bone? According to one of the foremost research experts in dietary fats and human health, Mary Enig, Ph.D., there's a case to be made for having as much as 50 percent of the fats in your diet as saturated fats for this reason. That's a far cry from the 7 to 10 percent suggested by mainstream institutions. If her reasoning is sound—and we believe it is— is it any wonder that the vast majority of women told to avoid saturated fat and to selectively use vegetable oils instead would begin to lose bone mass, develop osteoporosis, and get put on expensive prescription medications plus calcium to try to recover the loss in middle age?

- *Proper nerve signaling.* Certain saturated fats, particularly those found in butter, lard, coconut oil, and palm oil, function directly as signaling messengers that influence the metabolism, including such critical jobs as the appropriate release of insulin. And just any old fat won't do. Without the correct signals to tell the organs and glands what to do, the job doesn't get done or gets done improperly.

- *Healthy lungs.* For proper function, the airspaces of the lungs have to be coated with a thin layer of what's called lung surfactant. The fat content of lung surfactant is 100 percent saturated fatty acids. Replacement of these critical fats by other types of fat makes faulty surfactant and potentially causes breathing difficulties. Absence of the correct amount and composition of this material leads to collapse of the airspaces and respiratory distress. It's what's missing in the lungs of premature infants who develop the breathing disorder called infant respiratory distress syndrome. Some researchers feel that the wholesale substitution of partially hydrogenated (trans) fats for naturally saturated fats in commercially prepared foods may be playing a role in the rise of asthma among children. Fortunately, the heyday of trans fats is ending and their use is on the decline. Unfortunately, however, the unreasoning fear of saturated fat leads many people to replace trans fats with an overabundance of polyunsaturated vegetable oils, which may prove just as unhealthful.

- *Healthy brain.* You will likely be astounded to learn that your brain is mainly made of fat and cholesterol. Though many people are now familiar with the importance of the highly unsaturated essential fatty acids found in cold-water fish (EPA and DHA) for normal brain and nerve function, the lion's share of the fatty acids in the brain are actually saturated. (A diet that skimps on healthy saturated fats robs your brain of the raw materials it needs to function optimally.)

- *Strong immune system.* Saturated fats found in butter and coconut oil (myristic acid and lauric acid) play key roles in immune health. Loss of sufficient saturated fatty acids in the white blood cells hampers their ability to recognize and destroy foreign invaders, such as viruses, bacteria, and fungi. Human breast milk is quite rich in myristic and lauric acid, which have potent germ-killing ability. But the importance of the fats lives on beyond infancy; we need dietary replenishment of them throughout adulthood, middle age, and into seniority to keep the immune system vigilant against the development of cancerous cells as well as infectious invaders.

THE POTENTIAL BENEFITS
OF DIACYLGLYCEROL

While you're probably quite familiar with the term triglyceride, or triacylglycerol (TAG), as it's more correctly called in the medical research world, you may be less familiar with its close relative, diacylglycerol (DAG), which recent research has shown may be helpful in losing fat in and around the vital abdominal organs. Triglycerides—TAGs—are the main storage form of fat. The name connotes a structure—three fatty acid molecules (the *tri*) attached to a glycerol (sugar) backbone—and it's how the fats we eat and the fat stored around our middles, hips, and thighs are chiefly configured. When we eat a fat or oil, we absorb these TAGs into the blood. To get them inside the cells (to be stored or burned for energy), the body must disassemble them, chopping off the three fatty acid molecules from the backbone. The fatty acids then traverse the cell membrane and, on the other side, get immediately reassembled into TAGs once again.

In DAG, the glycerol backbone carries only two fatty acid strings on the three possible docking locations along its length (thus *di*glyceride, not *tri*glyceride). Exactly which two positions the fatty acid strings attach to—the first and second (so-called 1,2-DAG), the second and third (2,3-DAG), or the first and third (1,3-DAG)—changes the way the molecule behaves. The 1,3-DAG configuration hampers the process of reassembly on the far side of the membrane. Unable to reassemble properly, these fatty acids get shunted to the liver to be burned for energy instead of being stored.

Now for the translation. What this means for weight loss and, in particular, fat loss, has been the subject of intensive recent medical research. The upshot of that research suggests that in people trying to lose weight—especially fat inside the abdomen—replacing a portion of their daily intake of fats from other sources with fats rich in 1,3-DAG may be of great benefit. The benefits alluded to, at present, include better β-oxidation (fat burning), increased fat loss from both the subcutaneous (under the skin) fat stores and from the visceral (abdominal) fat stores, and improved blood sugar control. Possibly most important of all, the boost in β-oxidation has been shown in some research to clear fat out of the liver cells themselves, an important first step in rehabilitating the tendency to store fat in the middle body.

For this reason, especially in Weeks 1 and 2 of The Cure, you'll see a recommendation to add just a bit of Enova oil (a commercially available oil, high in 1,3-DAG) to your daily diet. To do so, you might choose to replace a little of the olive oil you use when making vinaigrettes for salads, replace a bit of cream in protein shakes, or use this oil in baking or other low-temperature (below 350° F) cooking. Be aware, however, that the oil isn't stable at higher heat; so do not use it for high-temperature frying.

THE DANGERS OF FRUCTOSE

There is possibly no food substance with more potential to harm—and to put fat into your liver and pounds around your waist—than fructose. Although you may be accustomed to thinking of fructose as "fruit sugar" and therefore as something wholesome and healthful, nothing could be further from the truth. While it's true that the simple sugar fructose was first isolated from fruit, there's actually not much of it in most fruits. Consequently, humans didn't eat huge amounts of fructose prior to the development of the sweetener derived from corn syrup, called high fructose corn syrup (HFCS).

Fructose is the substance routinely used to make laboratory animals obese and diabetic in order to study these disorders. It is deadly because of how it is metabolized by the body. It bypasses the normal regulatory points in the pathways that metabolize glucose, and as a result it is quickly turned to fat and stored in the liver and abdomen.

Since large quantities of HFCS (found in soft drinks, ice cream, cakes, cookies, candies, pastries, puddings, and in unlikely places such as salad dressings and ketchup) hit the market, human consumption of fructose has skyrocketed, and with it, the metabolic havoc it causes: insulin resistance, fatty infiltration of the liver, abdominal obesity, and diabetes—even among kids as young as 8 to 10 years old. Of all the food substances you should avoid to achieve and maintain a trim middle, added fructose heads the list.

WHY YOU SHOULD EAT ORGANIC AND NATURAL

The world has become laden with toxic chemical residues that find their way into the foods we eat. Since the advent of better living through chemistry, humans have released billions of tons of chemicals of one kind or another into the atmosphere or applied them to croplands to kill pests, stimulate crop growth, or produce goods. Consequently, conventionally grown produce is often heavily laden with pesticides and pollutants. Dairy farmers may feed their cows grain grown with the use of pesticides or may give their animals bovine growth hormones to increase milk production. In both cases, products from these chemically treated animals transfer their pesticide and/or hormone cargo to those who consume them.

Even though it may be a somewhat more expensive choice, we recommend buying organic and natural food products whenever possible. We advocate that you stretch your budget elsewhere to make room here. By doing so, you limit your exposure to numerous toxic substances. We say limit and not avoid because some amount of these toxic chemicals can even make it into cows raised on pastures never sprayed with any sort of chemical, because of the residues in the soil, in the ground water, and in the air. Once the substances are there, they don't go away; they accumulate in the earth, in plants, in animals that eat these plants, and in you. Even so, organic produce, organic dairy, and naturally raised meats offer the lowest possible toxic load. In dairy and meat, especially, the organic choice is important, since most of these chemical substances are fat soluble and will appear in the cream and the fat of the animal. Getting rid of the chemical load you now carry is difficult, but not impossible. We'll give you a method in Chapter 6, where we lay out Weeks 1 and 2 of The Cure.

EXERCISE DIFFERENTLY

On the "calories out" side of the energy balance equation, the energy spent every day by the body comes from several basic areas:

- *Basal metabolic rate (BMR).* The number of calories the body uses at complete rest, lying supine, upon first awakening, on an empty stomach. In sedentary people, BMR accounts for about 60 percent of total daily energy expenditure. The BMR is chiefly a function of lean body mass, which is why it behooves us to try to preserve our lean body mass as much as possible as we lose weight by eating sufficient protein, boosting leucine, engaging in weight-bearing (resistance) exercise, and by making sure that we take in sufficient iodine for optimal thyroid hormone function.
- *Thermogenic effect of food (TEF).* The energy cost of digesting, absorbing, and storing the food we eat. The TEF accounts for 10 to 15 percent of total daily energy expenditure.
- *Activity thermogenesis.* This consists of exercise activity thermogenesis (EAT) and non-exercise activity thermogenesis (NEAT), which is the energy we expend in sitting, standing, walking, talking, toe-tapping, playing the piano, pounding the computer keys—i.e., any movement that is not "officially" exercise. The NEAT can account for anywhere from 15 percent of total daily energy expenditure to as much as 50 percent in highly active people; fidgeting makes up a big portion of this difference.

The nutritional structure of The Cure encourages an increase in TEF, by virtue of its concentration on protein intake. Because protein has a higher TEF than carbohydrate, eating a diet replete with good protein reaps the reward of increased TEF. Additionally, a diet low in carbohydrate means that the body has to go to the trouble (read "spend calories") to turn protein into blood sugar. Moreover, a diet higher in quality fat increases the number of mitochondria (energy factories within the cells) and facilitates energy production and, when conditions merit, energy wasting. During times of low-carb calorie excess, these mitochondrial engines begin a process called futile cycling, which can "blow off" extra calories as heat. This phenomenon is a part of what explains the so-called metabolic advantage that occurs on a low-carb diet and may account for as much as 300 calories a day. The body's other means of expending extra low-carb calories is accomplished by adjusting its NEAT output. (A healthy diet structure will energize you and that energy will manifest itself in a desire to move.)

In our clinical practice, we've witnessed this phenomenon in action so often that it became expected. Overweight patients would come in complaining of no energy, of being too fatigued to do much of anything. Most physicians would counsel their patients to follow whatever dietary regimen they espoused and instruct them to join a gym, get out and walk, get some exercise. We didn't, because we realized that we didn't need to.

Once on a dietary structure that normalized their metabolic hormonal signals, their fat stores would open and make a huge number of calories available to them. When they did, they would no longer be tired and hungry, and the energy balance equation would be driven in the other direction, making the body *want* to spend calories. And with calories aplenty to spend, spontaneously, our patients would take up exercise of some sort: weight training, golf, line-dancing lessons, kickboxing classes, judo, kung fu, or karate. We could tell that it was about to happen because they would come into the clinic to weigh in with a spring in their steps, smiles on their faces, and a healthy glow about them. You will be able to see the same thing in yourself. Once accustomed to this new way of eating, you will find yourself not caring if there isn't a parking space at the door or that the elevator is full or that the moving sidewalk is shut down; the walk won't seem an imposition. You'll say yes to a dance or a swim or an invitation to go hiking or biking. And it's all because the energy balance equation is now free to move in both directions; calories are no longer on a one-way road to your fat cells, and your system is no longer stuck in "storage mode." You'll be free to move because you will now have access to the calories stored in your fat cells.

We'd be remiss if we didn't add that we are still big proponents of slow-speed strength training, just as we wrote about in *The Slow Burn Fitness Revolution* (Broadway Books, 2003). That's 30 minutes a week we recommend for an entirely different purpose we'll discuss shortly: building stronger muscles (and bones) and better muscle fitness. Be aware that sound scientific research has recently shown (again) that fat loss on a low-carb diet *without* exercise significantly exceeds fat loss on a low-fat, high-carb diet *with* exercise—even resistance exercise. And here's the really great news: adding resistance exercise to a low-carb diet can almost double the pounds of fat lost over just dieting. If you choose to add resistance exercise to The Cure, you will be amply rewarded, but even if you don't want to do so, take a look at one very simple thing you can do in the course of your day to specifically help trim your middle.

HARNESSING THE LAW OF LAPLACE

In the world of physics, the Law of Laplace states that the tension within the walls of a cylinder is greater than that in the walls of a sphere; and the larger the radius,* the greater the tension in the wall. It's easy to see this physical principle in action when you blow a soap

---

* The radius of a cylinder is the distance halfway across the cylinder from one wall to the other through the center.

bubble. The bubble comes out of the ring elongated, but quickly snaps into a perfect sphere; that's Laplace's law in action. The bubble seeks the configuration giving it the least possible tension in its delicate wall. The tension on the walls of a sphere is much less than that in a cylinder, allowing the bubble to survive a while. If you catch a bubble gently with your fingertip, it will often rest there intact, but if you press in slightly, you will change the configuration of the wall, increasing the tension beyond what the delicate soapy membrane can withstand, and pop! Your bubble is gone.

Or look at a sausage-shaped balloon. Once blown to its full capacity, the sidewalls are very tense where the balloon is the widest across and the walls are flat. As you move toward the two ends of the balloon, however, where the balloon tapers and becomes more rounded, the walls have more "give" in them, meaning the tension in the walls there is much less even though the pressure inside is exactly the same throughout the balloon. The Law of Laplace explains this difference in tension where the balloon is round.

What do a bubble, a balloon, and the Law of Laplace have to do with your middle-aged middle? Plenty, as it turns out, because the abdomen, unlike any other part of the body, is a soft-sided cylinder. It's easy to see the law in action. The arms and legs and neck are cylinders, but solid ones; increasing their girth may increase the tension in the wall, but there's nowhere for it to go. The chest cavity is a hollow cylinder and clearly expands and contracts, but it is bounded by the fairly immobile bony ribcage. Only the abdomen freely and quite visibly obeys the Law of Laplace, which can work for us or against us, depending on our relative girth.

As we gain abdominal weight and our waistlines expand, the Law of Laplace dictates that the tension across the abdominal wall must increase. To relieve the increased wall tension, the central abdomen pooches out, making a sphere of sorts—which we know as a potbelly or beer gut—with a smaller diameter and radius and thus lower tension. Dropping the wall tension takes a workload off the abdominal muscles.

You can harness the Law of Laplace to work in your favor by purposefully decreasing your girth in the middle with a simple maneuver. This "non-exercise activity" is a modern-day take on the ancient Hatha yoga practice called *nauli,* which the ancient teachings suggest stimulates the digestive fire, thereby removing toxic substances or indigestion and providing an internal cleansing to aid with excess phlegm, mucus, or fat. We can't attest to those particular results, but we're willing to agree that it sounds good. We like the maneuver, however, because it's an easy means of applying the Law of Laplace and tightening the radius of our middle-aged middles. We call it The Laplace in Place maneuver.

The beauty of this exercise is that it can be done anywhere: in the car at a stop light, in the line at Starbucks, standing at the stove or sink, waiting on your laundry to dry, riding the elevator, bus, or train, at your desk, on a park bench watching the kids swing, standing at the mirror shaving, while you're in the shower. Anywhere. Anytime. And each time that you do it, it entrains the muscles and tightens the radius and lowers the outward pressure.

THE CASE FOR BUILDING MUSCLE

Your muscle mass is a big part of what burns calories each day; remember your BMR is a function of it. Unfortunately, we lose ground with every tick of the biologic clock. Muscle mass peaks at about age 30, after which time the average person (male and female) loses about 1 percent of the body's muscle mass per year, unless he (or she) engages in muscle-building activities and eats a diet that supports muscle growth.

From an exercise standpoint, there is no better method of building muscle and bone than resistance exercise—for example, weight training. This principle is deeply ingrained in males from school age up, but not in women, who more often are the very ones who need to rebuild muscle and bone mass in middle age. Lately, light resistance training

TO PERFORM THE LAPLACE IN PLACE

Standing or sitting tall in your chair:

1. Inhale fully, completely filling your lungs to capacity.

2. As you slowly exhale, suck in your abdomen as if you were trying to touch your belly button to your spine. The key is to suck in hard, as hard as you can.

3. Once you feel tightness along your sides, try to hold this position for 10 seconds. (Over time, increase to 30 to 60 seconds.)

4. Exhale fully. This is one repetition.

5. Repeat twice. This is a set. Aim for at least 8 sets in the course of the day.

This single quick exercise may seem ridiculously simple and self-evident, and you may be tempted to discount its effectiveness. Doing so would be a mistake. The power of physical principles is at work here and the benefit to your middle will be enormous. Trust us; you will be sore from doing it. Real sore. If you still doubt the power, take a look at what one man achieved with no abdominal exercise other than this one.

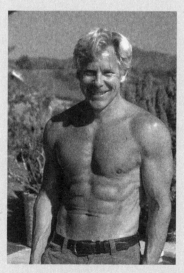

Mark Sisson, 55-year-old author of *The Primal Blueprint*.

for women has come into vogue, but that's not going to get the job done. To really build muscle takes more than endless repetitions of very low weights, which is how it is usually prescribed to women. It takes focused weight training, with significant weights, in repetitions that take the muscle under tension to complete failure. Many women resist this sort of training, fearing that it will cause them to develop bulky muscles. Rest assured it will not. Absent the input of lots of testosterone and other anabolic growth factors, women with balanced female hormone patterns will become strong and they will burn fat, but they will not bulk.

To achieve this end quickly, without spending hours and hours in the gym, we recommend the slow-speed, strength-training method. As mentioned previously, we co-authored a book on the subject with New York fitness guru Fred Hahn. If you're interested in gaining muscle mass and strengthening your middle-aged bones, and doing it in as little as 30 minutes a week, find a slow-speed strength trainer in your area or follow the guidelines in *The Slow Burn Fitness Revolution* (Broadway Books, 2003).

By learning to eat right and exercise differently, you can make giant strides toward whittling down your middle in a short space of time, strides that years of ELEM could never achieve. And best of all, you'll have mastered the tools that will let you keep your middle trim from now on.

5

TAKING SHAPE

"It is a capital mistake to theorize before you have all the evidence.
It biases the judgment."
—Sherlock Holmes,
in Sir Arthur Conan Doyle's *A Study in Scarlet*

What you weigh isn't as important as where your weight is; unfortunately, in middle age, it usually goes straight to the middle. We used the analogy more than a dozen years ago in *Protein Power* (as others have before and since) of pears and apples to represent the body shapes of those who carry their weight below the waist on the hips and thighs—the pears—and those who carry it in the middle, around the waist—the apples. Medical understanding that apple weight is more risky to health than pear weight isn't news, but the evidence indicting middle-body weight continues to pile up, and the reports still appear regularly on the front pages of newspapers and in headlines on the evening news.

Though it may be neither aesthetically pleasing nor particularly comfortable to carry too much body fat anywhere, you've learned that accumulation on the hips and thighs and elsewhere under the skin isn't as detrimental to health as fat stored in the middle, especially in and around the vital organs, the so-called visceral fat. This problem can afflict the overweight as well as seemingly normal-weight people.

Although it may seem paradoxical, it's quite possible—in fact, we've seen numbers of such cases in our many years of clinical practice—to be of normal weight, thin even, but carry excess fat inside the abdomen and not without consequence. Fat carried there is just as dangerous for normal-weight people as for overweight people, perhaps even more so. The thin 50-year-old woman with high blood pressure and high triglycerides often does not see her health problems as diet driven; rather, she sees it as an unfortunate reality for which she will take several prescription medications daily and keep on eating doughnuts. The 55-year-old man with six-pack abs won't usually connect his mild heart attack with fat he can't see. In our experience normal-weight people rarely grasp the need to change their eating habits and are often less likely than those who are overweight to recognize that their health concerns might stem from a metabolic problem (such as insulin-resistance-fueled accumulation of visceral fat) and do something about it nutritionally. Therefore, making some estimate of where your fat resides is a critically important step toward better health.

A WEIGHTY SUBJECT

There are various ways to assess weight. You can step on the scale and determine your weight in pounds, which you should certainly do, but with the understanding that the number you read on the scale doesn't tell the whole tale, since it doesn't give any information about what the weight is made of. Is it fat? Muscle? Fluid? The scale weighs them all. To refine the measurement of simple weight slightly, most insurers and government experts recommend using body mass index—the BMI—a ratio of weight and the mathematical square of the height in meters. Sounds fancy, but it likewise doesn't tell the whole story, since again it can't differentiate muscle from fat and can lead to some boneheaded conclusions about fitness or fatness. To wit, Arnold Schwarzenegger in his prime would have been classified as obese by the BMI tables, and he was veritably wasp-waisted. And The Governator isn't alone among muscular, fit celebrities whose BMIs classify them as over-weight or obese. Tom Cruise, Harrison Ford, Mel Gibson, Brad Pitt, and former President George W. Bush all find themselves in the same boat.*

There are skin calipers—little pincher devices used to measure the fat in various sites—on the back of the arm, over the shoulder blade, on the side of the waist—to determine how lean or fat a person is. This method does give an estimate of body-fat percentage for the average person, but still can be fooled by that thin person with little subcuta-neous (under the skin) fat who has too much fat inside the abdomen. Skin calipers don't really assess, even in those of us with plenty of sub-cutaneous fat, the truth of what lies within. And besides, calipers are notoriously difficult to use with accuracy, even by people who use them often. In fairness, however, Arnold and the other celebs mentioned above would have registered pretty healthy by this measure. None of them have much subcutaneous fat.

A further refinement, and the method we've always relied on, is to calculate the lean body mass and percentage of body fat, which can be estimated pretty closely using simple measurements, tables, and a for-mula, or can be done with minimally greater accuracy using a body fat analyzer—a computerized device that calculates fat percentage through bioimpedance measurements across the skin. This method does, at least, give a good estimate of overall fatness that's pretty easy to do and rea-sonably reliable. Home models of these devices have come on the mar-ket in recent years, so it's possible to make this kind of fat percentage measurement at home now, but the accuracy of the readout depends strongly on a person's state of hydration at the time and may be fraught with error. If you decide to use one of these devices, make sure to follow the manufacturer's instructions to the letter for reliable readings. But

* As reported on www.consumerfreedom.com/games.cfm/ID/1, referenced May 26, 2008.

these bioimpedance analyzers—even when used correctly—still don't differentiate abdominal fat from the fat under the skin.

The gold standard of fat measurement in medical studies has always been underwater weighing, but outside research labs it's impractical and unavailable to the average dieter. Even if you had an underwater weighing tank at home, however, it would still not answer the question you really need to know: how much of your fat is stored inside your abdomen?

In recent years, in medical and research settings, scientists have turned to computer X-ray technology (CT or EBT scans) to accurately calculate the volume of fat inside the abdomen. The CT and EBT can differentiate between the fat under your skin and the fat inside your abdomen with great accuracy, which is grand, but these are not methods you can apply at home and probably not even available at your doctor's office.

Recent research has given us a new tool using a measurement that found its genesis in CT scan technology. And with it, finally we can easily get a handle on what's inside. The measurement is called the Sagittal Abdominal Diameter, or SAD, and it's been shown in studies to be one of the best clinical correlates of visceral fat and of predicting health risks, including the risk of sudden death in men, even normal-weight ones. For this reason, we feel SAD to be the most critical measurement to make when you're battling the middle-aged bulge; it really tells the tale.

With a little ingenuity and a few simple items, you can use the method to make a SAD measurement right in your own home. Taking this measurement standing and lying flat and then figuring the difference between the two gives you a more accurate picture of how much fat is stored as VAT within the inner tube and how much is just beneath the skin.

Remember that the inner tube is bounded by a fairly thick wall of abdominal muscles that surround the visceral fat and prevent much change in its shape, whether you're standing or lying down. You can think of the abdominal muscular wall as being like a length of PVC pipe—standing on end or lying on its side, its shape and its diameter are constant. Conversely, nothing but skin contains the subcutaneous stores. This outer tube, more akin to a water balloon than a pipe, is much less rigid than the muscular wall. Therefore, when you stand, the fat beneath the skin acts like water under the influence of gravity; it seeks its own level, basically puddling around your waist in the typical "spare tire" configuration. A front-to-back measurement of your abdomen at its widest point, taken while standing, will yield a measurement of the full breadth of this spare tire. However, when you lie down, the sub-Q fat again flows like water, falling to the sides and, thus, the front-to-back measurement lying down will be a somewhat smaller one. If the numbers standing and lying are pretty close to the same, that indicates that a fair amount of fat is of the visceral type, bounded by the thick abdominal muscles, unable to move as freely as you change positions. And it also indicates that losing your middle-aged middle is much more important than cosmetic reasons alone would dictate.

This simple procedure gives you a realistic view of how much of your body fat resides inside your middle, where it can do you the most harm. And, better still, since taking the measurement is simple, it's easy to follow your progress as you make your way through the six weeks of The Cure and begin to dump fat from both the tubes.

MEASURING YOUR
SAGITTAL ABDOMINAL DIAMETER

In the research lab, scientists use a device called a slide beam abdominal caliper to measure the SAD of their study subjects. You can make your own homemade version of the device by using a pair of yardsticks or 18-inch rulers. It's helpful, though not required, to have a second person to assist you in making the measurement. (If you'd like, you can go to our website at www.6weekcure.com, where you can watch a video of exactly how to make this measurement.) To use the homemade version:

1. Lie on the floor on your back, knees drawn up, feet flat on the floor, to flatten your low back against the floor.

2. Lay one yardstick or ruler across your abdomen at what appears to be the widest point between the bottom tip of your breastbone and your belly button.

3. Stand the other yardstick or ruler on end beside your abdomen with the zero-inch end on the floor, in a position where the ruler can abut the end of the other ruler.

4. Read the height (in inches) where the bottom of the ruler lying across your abdomen hits the standing ruler.

5. This number is your lying SAD (L-SAD); record it in your Initial Assessment and Progress Log on page 285.

6. Now stand up against a wall, with your heels far enough from the wall that you can press your low back flat against the wall. Do not suck in your abdomen. Relax normally.

7. Place one ruler with its zero-inch end against the wall at your side at the widest point of your abdomen between the tip of your breast bone and your belly button.

8. Place the other ruler flat across your abdomen at about that same level.

9. Try to hold the rulers in place gently, without pressure.

10. Read the number on the ruler at your side, where the ruler across your abdomen meets it. Try to keep the two rulers perpendicular to each other to get a more accurate reading.

11. This number is your standing SAD (S-SAD); record it in your Initial Assessment and Progress Log on page 285.

The greater the difference between your standing and lying SAD measurements, the more likely it is that most of the middle-body fat is subcutaneous (SAT) fat—that is, mainly stored in the outer tube. The closer the two readings are together, the more likely it is that there is a significant amount of middle-body fat stored in and around the vital organs within the abdominal cavity—that is, visceral fat (VAT) in the inner tube. And, again, it is that fat that is most dangerous to your health. Fortunately on the right dietary scheme, middle-body fat, which is much more metabolically active, disappears quickly. You can track your progress in dumping inner-tube fat stores by repeating this calculation after Weeks 2, 4, and 6 as you progress through The Cure. Be sure to record your progress in your Initial Assessment and Progress Log.

THE MEASURE OF A MAN ... OR A WOMAN

To know where you want to go, it's helpful to know where you're starting. So get out your tape measure, dust off your scale, and sharpen your pencil. Here are the measurements you should make.

- *Weight.* Taken in the morning, just after awakening, after emptying your bladder, before you eat or drink, barefoot, naked or in light clothing, but whichever you choose, it should be the same each time you weigh yourself. There can be as much as a 2-pound difference in going barefoot or wearing shoes, in jeans and a jacket, or a tee-shirt and shorts, in a cotton nightshirt or a chenille bath robe. To be able to track your progress you need to strive for consistency. Fight down the urge to weigh more often than once a week, since day-to-day fluctuations in fluid balance (particularly in women) can undermine your apparent progress on the scale. Record your starting weight in your Initial Assessment and Progress Log.
- *Height.* Measure it, don't just write down what you think it is or what it's been in the past. Heights change gradually over time, usually in adulthood for the shorter. To measure, stand with bare feet flat on the floor, heels against a doorjamb, shoulders and back of head touching the jamb. Place a pencil on the top of your head, abutting the doorjamb and make a light mark. Then use a tape measure or yardstick to measure your height in inches from the floor to the mark. If you've had a height measurement taken at your doctor's

office in the last year, you can simply call them to get it. Record your height in your Initial Assessment and Progress Log.

- *Waist.* Take this measurement at belly-button level, with a tape measure laid gently against your skin, not pulled tightly or pinching it at all. The tape should be level to the ground, all the way around. For accuracy, take the measurement three times and average it—that is, add up the three measurements and divide by 3 to get an average waist circumference. Write the number in your Initial Assessment and Progress Log.

- *Hip measurement.* Take this measurement at the widest span around your hips to find the largest possible number between your hipbones and the start of your thighs. Try to keep the tape level with the floor all the way around. Again, average three readings and record.

- *Waist to hip ratio (WHR).* Now that you have these two critical measurements you can calculate the ratio that has remained a constant hallmark of youth and health across the millennia. To find your WHR, simply divide your waist measurement by your hip measurement. In women, a ratio of 0.7 is considered ideal. Above 0.85 signifies early metabolic trouble is brewing. In men a ratio of 0.8 to 0.9 is ideal; readings above 1.0 signal a need to take action. Record your ratio in your Initial Assessment and Progress Log.

WHAT YOUR DOCTOR OR LAB CAN TELL YOU

In addition to the basic anthropometric data above, you may want to get baseline readings on various health parameters, such as blood pressure, blood sugar, and lipids. While you may be using The Cure only to trim your middle, this dietary structure is also a powerful tool to correct and maintain control over a whole host of health issues that commonly afflict those in middle age and beyond (and sadly, nowadays, also those significantly younger). As long as you're going to spend the next six weeks getting trimmer, you might as well discover what a beneficial impact this eating plan is having on your underlying health. If you

AN IMPORTANT WORD OF CAUTION

Those of you who currently take prescription medications for fluid retention or lowering blood pressure, blood sugar, triglycerides, or cholesterol, particularly those that lower blood pressure or control blood sugar, take heed of the following information. This dietary structure works amazingly quickly to lower blood sugar and blood pressure. Nothing you have ever used to control these conditions will have prepared you for the response you are likely to get. The same may be true for your doctor. As a colleague of ours put it in a recent talk to physicians, "nothing in your medical experience will have prepared you for how quickly this therapy works." It is imperative that you work with your doctor as you begin this plan and keep a close watch on your readings, as he or she will need to be prepared to quickly taper and/or discontinue medications or your blood pressure or blood sugar could (and likely will) become dangerously low. If it does, you will find yourself examining the kitchen floor tiles from very close range. In our own practice, we halved or even stopped blood-sugar-lowering medications and most blood pressure medications on day one. **However, it is not safe to reduce or stop such medications on your own, so please enlist the aid of your health-care practitioner before you begin this powerful program!**

currently struggle with some of the so-called diseases of mid-life—diabetes, high cholesterol, high triglycerides, arthritis, or GERD—you should see these disorders dramatically improve in a very short space of time.

You'll see that your Initial Assessment and Progress Log has spaces provided to track the laboratory values that follow. These assessments aren't necessary for everyone, certainly not required to make the program work. The values, however, are the indicators of health and fitness that often become unhinged in middle age and that this program will correct. It's not just a slender middle that you'll be rewarded with by following the prescription we've outlined in The Cure, but also a healthier you.

METABOLIC MEASURES

- *Fasting glucose* (blood sugar).
- *Hemoglobin A1c*—a measure of average blood sugar over the previous 3 months.
- *Fasting insulin*—the easiest measure to detect hyperinsulinemia and insulin resistance, both strongly tied to accumulating fat in the liver and in the abdominal area.
- *High sensitivity TSH (hs-TSH)*—a test that measures a brain hormone produced to stimulate the thyroid gland (one of the body's most important metabolic regulators). When the value is high, this means the brain is not detecting enough thyroid action and is calling for the release of more thyroid hormone. Elevated TSH doesn't speak about the cause for the lack of action, which may require further testing to determine if the thyroid gland is underproducing, if the body is making antibodies against the thyroid hormone or against the gland, or any of a number of other reasons.
- *Iodine saturation percentage*—iodine is among the most essential elements for proper functioning of the metabolism. The thyroid hormone—the lynchpin of metabolic drive—requires four molecules of iodine, without which the output of thyroid hormone drops and the metabolism slows down. But the need for iodine goes beyond the thyroid gland; many other body tissues require it as well. In generations past, before iodine was added to table salt, people (and even livestock) living in areas with iodine-poor soil were subject to the development of an iodine deficiency disorder called goiter, a usually benign enlargement of the thyroid gland. Iodizing salt vastly reduced the incidence of goiter, but the addition of the type of iodine put into table salt doesn't always do the trick for the many other tissues that rely on this element for proper function and sometimes, body stores

fall low. Estimates are that 90 percent of Americans are low in the types of iodine they need for good health and optimal metabolic function. This simple test to determine whether your stores of iodine are adequate involves collecting a urine specimen, taking a prescribed number of iodine pills, and collecting all urine for the next 24 hours to obtain another specimen. See the Resources for where your physician can obtain this test for you.

- *Liver enzymes*—enzymes are molecules that facilitate chemical reactions, and the liver is full of them. Normally, the enzymes inhabit the interior of the cells in which they're made and a small and fairly stable amount of them make it into the bloodstream. If the liver cells are injured by something—medication, excess alcohol, hepatitis infection, or accumulation of fat droplets within them—the enzymes within them (primarily two, known as AST and ALT) leak out and their higher levels in the blood can be detected and reported as elevated liver enzymes. Having normal liver enzyme levels doesn't mean you don't have fat accumulation in your liver, but having elevated ones may mean you really need this program! Fortunately, except in the case of hepatitis, of course, you'll quickly see a return to normal levels after just a few short weeks on a good dietary structure.

CARDIOVASCULAR MEASURES

- *Total cholesterol, HDL, LDL, and triglycerides* are the blood fats commonly viewed as risk factors for heart disease. To our minds, the only two important ones are triglycerides and HDL. The most meaningful lipid value predictor of heart disease risk is clearly the ratio of triglycerides divided by HDL. A number over 5 warns of increased risk; a number below 5 is a good sign, and the further below, the better. As to total cholesterol numbers, even in people with extreme levels of cholesterol (those with the genetic disorders of hypercholesterolemia, for example, who may commonly run levels in 400 to 600 mg/dl range), the incidence of heart attack is not worse than in people with lower numbers, making it questionable to worry about total cholesterol or LDL. The exception would be in people with a small dense LDL pattern, which does appear to be associated with heightened cardiovascular risk. Determining particle size (small dense LDL versus large, fluffy LDL) requires a specialized test called a gel electrophoresis. Particle size, however, varies inversely with triglyceride levels, making the triglyceride reading a good surrogate marker for this reading: high triglycerides, small particle size; low triglycerides, large particle size. The common practice of putting everybody on a statin who has an LDL reading over 120 or a cholesterol over 200 is insanity. That's particularly true for women, in whom not a single shred of evidence exists that lowering cholesterol with a statin does any good whatsoever. Moreover, cholesterol is a molecule of critical importance, produced by the liver, the gut, and every single cell in the body. If it were the evil you've probably been led to believe it to be, why would every cell in the body produce it? We've written extensively on this topic in previous books, filling entire chapters, and on our blogs. If you wish to know more, go to www.proteinpower.com/drmike and search the term "cholesterol."

- *Apolipoprotein-B (Apo-B)* is the main constituent of LDL (the low-density lipoprotein or so-called bad cholesterol), making up nearly 90 percent of the particle. It functions to make cholesterol (a waxy, water-repellant alcohol) soluble within the blood, boosting LDL's cholesterol transport capacity to the tissues. Many authorities feel that Apo-B is a better marker for heart disease risk than cholesterol; in fact, recent research suggests that it can also be a good indirect method of assessing LDL particle size. Like triglyceride levels, Apo-B is another bargain-priced surrogate for gel electrophoresis to determine the particle size of LDL. Checking the Apo-B as well as the LDL can tell you volumes about your real cardiovascular wellness and help you fend off well-meaning but misguided entreaties to take a statin drug. Since every LDL molecule is mainly made of Apo-B, it's a good estimation of particle number. Thus, if the LDL reading stays the same or even goes up, but the Apo-B goes down, you know that you have fewer particles. Even though the value reads the same or higher, it's not because there are more LDL particles, but rather because the particles are bigger; they're the large and fluffy (harmless) type, and that's a good thing for your cardiovascular well-being. If the LDL goes down but the Apo-B goes up (as happens sometimes on a low-fat, high-carb diet) it's actually a bad sign, since more Apo-B means more LDL particles and the lower reading means those particles are of the small, dense (much more atherogenic and dangerous) type.

- *Lipoprotein(a) [Lp(a)]*—levels of this substance are to some extent genetically determined. It binds to other more commonly known lipoproteins (LDL and HDL) and rides along to the lining of the arteries, where it interferes with the body's ability to dissolve blood clots. High levels (above about 30 mg/dl) increase risk of heart disease by thirty times. The little-known fact is that although Lp(a) elevation rarely responds to the standard "healthy heart diet," research indicates that there is one food substance that will reduce it: saturated fat.

- *Ferritin*—a molecule that is the storage form of iron in your body. People with middle-body fat and/or other components of the metabolic syndrome tend to accumulate excess iron, which can impair the normal function of glands, such as the thyroid, and increase the risk of heart damage in the event of a heart attack. During times of illness, the body hides iron from invading germs in the ferritin stores, so it's important not to take this test if you are or have been sick, even with a cold. Ferritin is the reservoir of iron the body calls upon in the event of blood loss to make new blood cells, so having an appropriate amount—10 to 50 mg/ml—is important. Although the normal range reported by most laboratories will be much higher, metabolic research suggests that ferritin levels over 50 indicate metabolic iron storage disorder and a need to get rid of some of it. The method for doing that is to call your local blood bank and make an appointment to give blood. About a month later, recheck your ferretin level and if it's still too high, in another month or two, give again. Regularly giving blood often improves metabolism and boosts weight loss—and not just from the weight of the blood. (See the discussion in Chapter 6.)

- *High-sensitivity C-reactive protein (hs-CRP)*—a measure of inflammation. It's quite unspecific, meaning if it's elevated it doesn't tell you what's going on, just that something of an inflammatory nature is happening within the body. But even that information is helpful because most of the diseases of middle age have at least some inflammatory component driving them, even obesity and heart disease. If this value is elevated—and it often is in people with metabolic syndrome—you should expect to see a nice drop by the time you've completed The Cure.

CORTISOL AND THE SEX HORMONES

As you learned in Chapter 2, chronic stress and lack of sleep can cause an increase in the hormone cortisol, your body's stress hormone, designed by nature to be released in ebbs and flows during the 24-hour cycle and only intermittently to assist in times of crisis. Aging causes a gradual decline in the gender-specific hormones of reproduction, mainly estrogen and progesterone for women and primarily testosterone for men. Laboratory evaluation of these hormones has now become simple, though not inexpensive, unless your physician orders the tests and your insurance covers the cost. We recommend testing the levels of these hormones in saliva, since that is a measure of "free hormone" available to do its job and it's painless. (See Resources for where you or your physician can obtain laboratory test kits for home collection.)

- *Cortisol*—the body's stress hormone. Its level fluctuates during the day and night. The pattern of fluctuation can give important clues to what's going on in that system. Home collection (the saliva test kit mentioned above) is by far the most convenient method for the patient, since gauging the pattern means a collection first thing in the morning, at noon, in the evening, and at bedtime, a scheduling nightmare for getting blood drawn at a clinic or laboratory.

- *Estrogen (estradiol, estriol, estrone)*—three types of estrogen that occur in varying levels throughout the reproductive life of women. The rise in estrogens at puberty promotes "feminine fattening" in the pelvic abdomen, hips, and thighs through the peak of female reproductive life. Paradoxically, it is the decline in estrogens (primarily in estradiol) in mid-life and beyond that fuels fat storage in the middle. In order to effectively trim middle-body fat, some women may require hormone replacement therapy—of the right kind—to normalize these levels. For decades, the drug most commonly prescribed to treat the symptoms of menopause was Premarin, a prescription estrogen replacement heavy in estrone, derived from the urine of pregnant mares, hence the name. The balance of estrogen types in Premarin isn't remotely like the balance in human females and rare, in our experience, was the woman prescribed this drug who didn't bemoan a 20- to 40-pound weight gain. Addressing the decline with the wrong kind of hormonal replacement only compounds the problem, leading to the accumulation of more middle-body pounds. To reap the benefits of safe estrogen replacement without the specter of weight gain, we have for many years recommended using the smallest effective amount of bio-identical estrogens—usually estradiol or a combination of estriol and estradiol to reverse this imbalance.
- *Progesterone*—a hormone best known as the protector of the uterus in counterpoint to estrogen's actions.* It is also quite important in

---

* Estrogen causes buildup and growth of the lining of the uterus. Unopposed, it increases the risk of uterine cancer. Progesterone serves to counteract this risk, protecting the uterus (and breasts, too, for that matter) from the proliferative effects of estrogen. Men, too, may benefit from replacing a small amount of this hormone (they don't have much, but need some) as studies suggest that it exerts a protective counterpoint against the proliferative effects of testosterone and may protect the prostate from enlargement or cancer.

normalizing fat distribution and in building bone mass. Many clinicians (ourselves among them) feel progesterone is more important than estrogen for overall good health. When progesterone levels are found to be low, successful fat loss can be difficult. If you have low levels, consider replacing the hormone—again with a bio-identical topical cream—to restore levels to those of a young healthy individual.

- *Testosterone*—for men in their middle years, waning levels can result in lean body (muscle) wasting, loss of libido, depression, sleep disturbances, and a potbelly. Replacement to correct the levels to those of a healthy younger man may prove beneficial in rehabilitating the body's frame and trimming the middle.

MARTI'S STORY

Marti was frustrated. She'd just endured a lengthy, finger-wagging lecture by her internist about her elevated cholesterol. "Your cholesterol is still 240 and your LDL is up, too; you need to go on a statin," he told her for about the seventh time in as many years. "You've tried diet and exercising and your LDL and total cholesterol are still up there," he'd said.

But Marti steadfastly refused him, again. "I'm down from the 280 it was five years ago," she offered. "I'll work harder on my diet and I'll try to exercise more. It's been tough this year because of my knee." She had fallen, hiking, and twisted her knee, tearing her ACL, the central stabilizing ligament. The injury left her with a very unstable knee, which over the years had resulted in wear and tear on the cartilage. In the last year, it had become a painful, unstable knee.

"Six months," he'd replied, "and if it's not down, you've simply got to take the statin."

Marti was not a fan of drugs and their potential side effects. For years, she had tried to eat less fat, limit eggs, and focus on whole natural foods, and she had bought and taken every natural remedy she could lay her hands on to get her cholesterol down, all with only modest success. She'd even tried a low-carbohydrate approach, which had improved her numbers to where they were now. Over dinner with friends one evening a few months later, Marti heard about The Cure from someone who was following the plan, and she decided to give diet one more shot. She contacted us and we got her started.

After following just the first two weeks of The Cure, she telephoned us one morning, positively giddy with excitement. She'd been to have her blood drawn, the results were in, and her cholesterol numbers were amazing. Her total cholesterol had dropped to 174. Everything was better: her triglycerides were under 100, her HDL was over 60, her ratios were improved in every way. And she'd lost 8 pounds in two weeks! She couldn't believe it and neither could her physician.

"Are you taking medication?" he inquired.

"No, nothing."

"Exercising more?"

"Not exercising at all, right now. The knee, remember?"

"This is astonishing. What did you do?"

So she filled him in on her new regimen, left the office, and immediately phoned us from her car to share her delight. "Dr. Eades," she said, "you just don't understand. I've been working on this for seven years. Seven years! I don't know how to thank you."

Marti's story exemplifies something that we have preached for decades: food—the right food—is the most powerful medicine of all. It is results like these, not atypical at all in our practice, that make us encourage you to check your numbers before you begin and after you've completed your plan. You, too, will be amazed at the incredible improvement this program will make, not just in your girth but in all the indicators of metabolic health and disease. Remember, a thin midsection is associated with health, so it makes sense that bringing your belly to more youthful proportions restores other indicators of health as well.

And remember, nothing in your experience will have prepared you for how quickly this plan works.

PART 2

6

THE CURE: WEEKS 1 AND 2

"How long does getting thin take?"
—*Winnie the Pooh,* (A. A. Milne)

The cure for your middle-aged middle can't begin until you get the lynchpin of the metabolism—your hard-working liver— back in top-notch condition. As you learned in Chapter 2, a lifetime of dietary excess, junk food, overindulgence in alcohol and caffeine, and popping pills—whether the over-the-counter variety for everything from headaches and sports injuries to arthritic joints or daily prescription medications for elevated blood pressure and cholesterol— takes its toll and leaves the liver struggling to do all the many jobs it must do to keep the metabolism humming along smoothly. So the first order of business must be to take the stress off the liver and quickly set the stage, nutritionally, for the liver cells to dump the fat that crowds their interiors and disrupts their function. This is Job One, because fat in the liver leads to fat in the middle.

Turning around the forces that drive you to store fat in your middle takes some commitment and effort. The prescription may seem tough at first glance, but the duration of the effort is short and the payoff to your metabolic balance is enormous. In our experience (with ourselves and with patients), the best, fastest, most effective, and ultimately least painful method is just to suck it up and do it all the way. Like jumping into cold water, it's a task best done quickly and with purpose, not an inch at a time. So if you're ready, let's jump in.

THE RULES OF THE GAME—WEEKS 1 AND 2

1. No alcohol whatsoever. Much as we love our beer, wine, and spirits (and believe us when we say that we do), a brief break from imbibing will do a world of good for your liver. Although there are some real health benefits, which we'll get into a bit later, from a moderate intake of alcohol, especially wine, you must remember that alcohol is also a toxic compound, a delicious poison of sorts. And, as such, it must be "detoxified." As is true for most toxic substances, the liver serves as the main detoxifying organ, which means that when you drink alcohol, it makes extra work for an already struggling system. Alcohol is also a compound that is quickly and easily converted to triglycerides (or fat droplets) by the liver, meaning yet more work. Worse still, in short order, those fat droplets accumulate within the liver cells. Since your job at this point in The Cure is to focus on getting the fat out of the liver, not putting more in, we recommend abstinence—no booze—in Weeks 1 and 2.

2. No caffeine whatsoever. For us, since we drink a lot of coffee every day, this is a hard one, but again, it is important in the early going. Just as with alcohol, there are actually a number of important benefits from moderate caffeine use that we'll cover shortly, but because the liver must handle the caffeine, drinking coffee, caffeinated sodas, and black or green tea means more work for it to do. The middle-aged liver becomes less and less capable of handling caffeine, which then hangs around in the bloodstream, unhandled, for longer, able to exert its stimulating effects. This phenomenon explains why, at some point, many

TAPERING OFF CAFFEINE

An easy way to reduce your caffeine intake is to mix your full-strength coffee (tea or cola beverage) half and half with a decaffeinated version for a couple of days. Then mix one part full caf with two parts decaf for a couple of days. Then mix one part caf with three parts decaf for a couple of days. Then mix one part caf with four parts decaf. By the end of the week, you'll be off caffeine.

Another option is to drink espresso, which contrary to its high-octane reputation has only about half the caffeine per single serving as drip, perked, or pressed coffee. Going from drip to espresso or café Americano (hot water plus espresso) instantly cuts your caffeine load in half. From there you can move to half-caf espresso and then to decaf espresso. If you're a coffee lover, you'll be delighted with the full-bodied taste of decaf espresso versus the drip stuff. If you're unfamiliar with café Americano, visit any Starbucks or your favorite coffee bar, where you'll find it on the menu. Or visit our website at www.proteinpower.com to find a YouTube video in the Dr. Michael Eades's blog archives, demonstrating how to make your own Americano at home.

adults as they enter middle age begin the shift away from caffeinated beverages, first late at night, then after dinner, then late in the afternoon, then finally altogether. Sleeplessness from caffeine is almost *de facto* proof of a liver in need of a rest.

If you consider yourself a real caffeine junkie, you might want to spend a pre-start week—a Week 0, let's call it—tapering off your caffeine intake instead of going cold turkey, which can give you a throbber of a caffeine withdrawal headache.* For tips on how to do that, see the sidebar on "Tapering off Caffeine."

---

* Occasionally people will experience a headache from caffiene withdrawal or an increase in the by-products of fat burning during the first few days of the diet. If you do, and drinking more water doesn't help, you may take a couple of regular-strength aspirin—if absolutely necessary and if you tolerate aspirin.

3. *No unnecessary medications.* Take no medications, particularly such products as acetaminophen (Tylenol), ibuprofen (Advil, Motrin), or other NSAIDS, unless prescribed by your doctor, as these medications adversely impact the liver. In the sidebar that follows you'll find a list of common medications (both prescription and over-the-counter) that are especially hard on the liver. Avoid taking any of them during the first week or two on the program unless deemed necessary by your physician. Even then, we recommend that you discuss with your doctor the possibility of taking a break from these and other liver-toxic medications for a few weeks to let your liver take a breather. Obviously, if you must keep taking any of these medications, do so; never discontinue prescription meds without your doctor's express consent and supervision. If absolutely necessary, for pain or fever, try two regular-strength aspirin, which has less effect on the liver.

3. *Follow the simple "3-and-1" food plan.* Here's your roadmap to optimal weight-loss nutrition: drink your choice of any of the tasty and filling, nutrition-packed Power Up! Protein Shakes (basic recipe on page 115) three times each day. Eat one of the richly satisfying food meals prescribed for Weeks 1 and 2 each day. Three shakes and a meal—that's the 3-and-1 plan. Nothing could be simpler.

We've specifically designed the meals to create the proper metabolic hormone environment and provide plenty of the particular kinds of amino acids, fats, and micronutrients you should be eating to promote liver recovery. Your prescribed meal can be eaten at breakfast, lunch, or dinner (we've given you multiple options for each) so that the plan is flexible enough to fit with your schedule and lifestyle.

Although for these first two weeks you may eat a "real" food meal only once a day, you make the call on any given day as to when that will be. For instance, if you love to eat a big breakfast on Saturday or Sunday morning, then by all means stick to your routine and enjoy one of the breakfast options on either or both of those days, and then follow it with Power Up! Protein Shakes at lunch, dinner, and as a snack. If eating lunch is something you must often do in the course of your work, you

DRUGS THAT MAY CAUSE LIVER DYSFUNCTION OR DAMAGE

The liver is the main organ responsible for detoxifying a host of drugs so that they can be safely removed from the body. This list contains the drugs most commonly known to put toxic stress on the liver, but it is by no means exhaustive. Check with your pharmacist or physician if you take medications that may damage the liver.

acetaminophen
  (Tylenol)

acebutolol

actinomycin D

adrenocorticosteroids
  (cortisone)

allopurinol

amoxicillin/clavulanate
  (Augmentin)

anti-thyroid drugs

atenolol

azathioprine

captopril

carbamazepine

carbimazole

cephalosporins (Keflex,
  Ceclor)

chlordiazepoxide

cholorpropamide

cloxacillin

cimetidine (Tagamet)

cyclophosphamide

cyclosporine

danazol

dantrolene

diazepam

diclofenac

diltiazem

diospyramide

enalapril

enflurane

erythromycin

ethambutol

ethionamide

flurazepam

flutamide

glyburide ?

gold

griseofulvin

haloperidol

halothane

ibuprofen

indomethacin

isoniazid

ketoconazole

labetalol

mainserin

maprotiline

mercaptopurine

methotrexate

methyltestosteron

metoprolol

naproxen

nicotinic acid

nifedipine

nitrofurantoin

NSAIDs

oral contraceptives

oxacillin

penicillins

penicillamine

phenelizine

phenindione

phenobarbital

phenothiazines

phenylbutazone

phenytoin

piroxicam

probenecid

pyrazinamide

quinidinequinine

ranitidine

salicylates

sulfonamides

sulindac

tamoxifen

tetracyclines

thiabendazole

tolbutamide

tricyclic antidepressants

valproic acid

verapamil

may choose instead to make lunch your food meal when needed, with Power Up! shakes for breakfast, dinner, and a snack. If sitting down to dinner with the family is an important part of your life, drink your shakes for breakfast, lunch, and a snack, and then enjoy dinner with the family as your prescribed meal. Remember, this pattern of eating will only last for two weeks.

As to the meals themselves, if there is something on the menu for a given meal that you simply can't or won't eat, review the lists of equivalent substitutions in the Food Substitutions Lists in the Appendix. To make an exchange, simply find the food item you wish to omit and substitute one of the other items on its list.

We've designed this nutritional structure with two specific goals in mind. First, it's easy to follow, straightforward, and eliminates all the guesswork about what to eat. Second, by weighting the diet heavily with quality protein—especially protein sources rich in the branched-chain amino acids—but keeping the number of calories relatively low, we set the stage for your maximal rate of abdominal fat loss in this first week and the next, while preserving your lean muscle tissue. Fat loss in this region comes not only from fat stored *around* the organs, which begins to pare down the middle immediately, but also from fat *within* the organs, which means emptying the fat droplets out of the liver cells, your main goal of the week. Plenty of protein, in the absence of lots of calories or carbohydrates, also serves as an important reservoir the body can use to produce blood sugar at a slow, steady rate, which helps to keep hunger at bay.

4. Take important supplemental nutrients. We've designed a regimen of supplemental micronutrients that specifically meet the metabolic demands that occur as you begin the program (see sidebar). This prescribed regimen will replace critical electrolytes and minerals, such as potassium, magnesium, and calcium, that the body may lose at a greater rate during this metabolic switchover period; it will boost levels of iodine and iodide, which are substances clinical testing has found to be low in 90 percent of tested subjects and critical to normal metabolism (see discussion in Chapter 5); and it will support the liver, boost fat burning, preserve lean tissue, and provide all nutrients necessary for optimal general health. Replacing lost potassium is critical in the first two weeks of The Cure. Magnesium helps to maintain the potassium balance, so look for a product that contains both in near equal amounts—aim for about 400 mg of each one (that's usually four of the 99 mg over-the-counter-strength tablets available at most vitamin shops or grocery stores*). We implore you to heed this advice; unless you replenish the potassium you'll lose every day in this first two weeks as you lose fat and shed excess retained fluid, you may become very tired and could suffer muscle cramping or even heart rhythm disturbances. It's seriously important, so we repeat: take your potassium.

5. Substitute a tablespoon of the oil you usually use with a tablespoon of DAG oil.† Medical research has shown that supplementing your diet with DAG oil may assist in the fat-burning process, especially of abdominal fat. You can mix a teaspoon of the oil into your shakes, add it to salad dressings, or just take a spoonful, like medicine. In our experience, it's best to take the oil in small, divided doses as recommended here—that is 1 teaspoon three times a day. Although some people tolerate it well, others will experience mild nausea if they take too much at once.

6. Drink water or caffeine-free, water-based beverages daily when you are thirsty. Remember that you will lose some fluid as insulin falls in these first two weeks, and replacing it is important. Additionally, in our experience with many thousands of patients, those who drink plenty of water seem to lose weight better. Why this would be the case we're not entirely sure, but perhaps it has to do with increasing the loss of ketone bodies (which contain calories, after all) via the urine.

---

* If you currently take any blood pressure medication, consult with a pharmacist or doctor first.

† DAG stands for diacylglycerol, an oil sold as Enova in grocery stores.

SUPPLEMENTAL NUTRIENTS FOR WEEKS 1 AND 2

Select a basic supplement providing, *at minimum*, the RDI of the following nutrients:

Vitamin A	5000 IU
Vitamin C	60 mg
Vitamin D3	400 IU
Vitamin E	30 IU
Vitamin K	80 mcg
Thiamin	1.5 mg
Riboflavin	1.7 mg
Niacin	20 mg
Vitamin B6	2 mg
Folate	400 mcg
Vitamin B12	6 mcg
Biotin	3000 mcg
Pantothenic Acid	10 mg
Calcium	1000 mg
Phosphorous	1000 mg
Iodine	148 mcg
Magnesium	400 mg
Zinc	15 mg
Selenium	70 mcg
Copper	2 mg
Manganese	2 mg
Chromium	120 mcg
Molybdenum	75 mcg
Potassium	99 mg × 4

continued

Supplements specific to improving liver funtion:

Silymarin (milk thistle)	200 mg
Alpha lipoic acid	100–300 mg
Coenzyme Q10	60–300 mg
Magnesium	400 mg
Potassium	400 mg

7. Get a good night's sleep—aim for at least 7 hours every night. You learned about the importance of sleep in Chapter 2. We suggest you follow this recommendation for all six weeks of The Cure and thereafter.

8. Add some salt. Although it may sound like heresy, to help keep your fluid balanced you might actually need to replace some lost sodium (salt) during this first two weeks. You'll know if that's the case if you feel a little light-headed upon standing or a little winded with exercise. When insulin falls, the kidney releases sodium along with potassium, which can take some fluid with it and drop blood pressure—occasionally a little too much. Adding a bit of salt back into the diet can help restore fluid balance to normal. To do so, you may salt your food with quality salt (Celtic Sea Salt is our favorite for its good mineral profile) or eat a dill pickle half once or twice a day. If you like it, you can even drink a little pickle juice or boullion.

9. Add D-Ribose. This is an optional recommendation if you are physically active, work out with weights, engage in demanding recreational activities, or work at a physically demanding job. If so, add about 2500 mg of the special sugar called D-ribose (available at health food stores and online) to your shakes each day. D-ribose provides quick muscle energy without raising insulin levels. It also helps to prevent soreness after the workout.

ONE LAST MEASURE

There's one additional measure you can take to rid yourself of some of the toxic compounds that are stored in fat: give blood. Pesticides, growth factors, hormones, medications, and pollutants of all sorts, which come into the body through the foods we eat, the water we drink, and the air we breathe, become trapped in our fat tissues. As we liberate fat through weight loss or simply by fasting between meals, these stored substances enter in the bloodstream, where they hang out for a bit only to be reabsorbed and restored in the fat, accumulating over time. Many of these substances are believed to disrupt normal endocrine and metabolic function, making it ever more difficult to lose weight as we age.

At the end of your first two weeks on The Cure, you will be mobilizing fat maximally, and that is the prime time to rid yourself of some of this toxic load. To do this, go to your local blood bank and give a unit of whole blood. If you're a male or a female who has never been pregnant,* ask to give a unit of packed red blood cells and two units of plasma (a procedure called an *apheresis*), and get rid of twice as much of the load. The substances liberated from your fat mobilization will be contained in the liquid portion of your blood (your plasma); therefore, by giving a unit of whole blood or a unit of red blood cells and double plasma, you will both be doing something good for yourself and benefiting those who need blood or blood products urgently. Don't fear that

---

* There is a rare disorder called Transfusion Related Acute Lung Injury (TRALI) that occurs in people who *receive* blood products (plasma, platelets, clotting factors). It seems to occur more commonly when they receive plasma from women who have been pregnant (which is a lot of women), and thus the federal oversight agencies in charge have banned collecting plasma via apheresis (machine separation of the plasma from the red blood cells) from this group of women.

you'd be giving toxic substances to the recipient of your blood; all blood given by anyone in this day and age contains these substances, since all people living in industrialized countries have been liberally exposed to all manner of toxic compounds throughout the bulk of their lives. Remember, too, that at a time of emergency, human blood is a lifesaving fluid that can't be manufactured, except by humans.

Giving blood is something that you can do only about once every two months at most, although you can give plasma more frequently. Certain conditions and medical history preclude giving blood at all,* at least if it's to be donated for use by another person. Whether you choose to donate every two months (which you certainly don't have to do), or do it less often—say, twice or three times a year, as we generally do—always precede it with several days of focused dieting (such as the structure of Weeks 1 and 2 of The Cure). You'll help break the accumulation cycle of those environmental substances that can throw a monkey wrench into your metabolic machinery in middle age.

To maximize the benefit to you (in removing stored poisons), fast overnight and don't eat anything before the donation. Do, however, drink a cup of caffeinated coffee or tea (or a caffeine-stoked sugar-free energy drink, such as Sugar Free Rock Star or Low Carb Monster). The caffeine helps to mobilize fat and will further enhance the results of your donation in removing toxic substances. Be sure to take a healthy snack with you to eat *after* you've donated, so as to restore your blood sugar, because the blood banks only offer empty carbs in the form of cookies, cheese nips, whole-grain chips, and granola bars that have the nutrient profile of a Snickers bar. You don't need that junk; you need *water* to restore your fluid level, maybe a little *salt* to keep it there, and something *decent* to eat. Take a protein shake in a thermos or a couple

---

* People with certain medical disorders or on certain medications cannot give blood at the volunteer blood banks. The blood bank will screen for these problems. These people can, however, undergo phlebotomy (giving blood) at their physician's office, if he or she is willing to perform it for them. Some physicians will, others will not.

of hard-boiled eggs, some salami slices, and several dill pickles or perhaps some beef jerky and nuts. Whatever you do, don't let the blood bank's misguided good intentions put a crimp in your dietary plans.

PRESCRIBED MEALS TO MANAGE
YOUR MIDDLE-AGED MIDDLE

Three times a day, every day, for the first two weeks you should drink a Power Up! Protein Shake. Depending on your likes and dislikes, you can flavor the shakes to suit your fancy—say, a Wild Berry in the morning, a Caramel Cappuccino at noon, and a Turtle Sundae in the afternoon. See the box for the basic recipe that we use ourselves, followed by a host of flavor recipes to tempt your taste buds.

Every component in the Power Up! Protein Shakes is there for a reason; each plays an important role in pushing the metabolism in the direction you want it to go. We designed the shake formula to maximize visceral abdominal fat loss, preserve lean muscle, keep insulin controlled, and boost cellular energy stores to keep you well fed at the cellular level, which keeps you hunger free. If you get into a time bind, just a quick mix of a commercial protein shake and some water is better than eating the wrong things, but adhering to our shake formula will maximize your progress.

ADD AN EGG?

Research has shown that, during weight loss, people (especially women) mobilize abdominal fat stores better with the addition of a foodstuff that may surprise you: cholesterol. Nowadays, you're used to hearing doctors admonish people to cut back on cholesterol in foods, to eat the whites of eggs but not the yolks, and to look for "cholesterol free" on a label as assurance of the product's healthfulness, but there's really no evidence—zero, zip, *nada*—to support this onerous advice. There is no evidence, in fact, to tie the intake of dietary cholesterol to the level of

BASIC POWER UP! PROTEIN SHAKE

1 serving

¾ cup (6 ounces) cold water

1 packet Splenda, stevia, xylitol, or erythritol sweetener (optional)

2 tablespoons heavy cream (organic, if possible) or premium coconut
  milk

Flavorings, as desired (see pages 118–119)

1 to 3* scoops low-carb whey protein (any flavor)

2500 mg leucine (in branch-chain amino acid supplement capsules or
  powder)†

2500 mg D-ribose powder (optional)

Approximately 1 cup ice cubes

Place all the ingredients in a blender in the order above and blend on high
speed until smooth. Adjust the amount of ice to achieve preferred consistency.
Drink immediately.

Note: You can also make a thinner version of the shake by shaking ingredients
in a tightly sealed, lidded container if no blender is available. The ice will chill
the shake, but won't be crushed to make it thick.

---

* The amount of protein in these products varies. Most contain 18–22 grams per scoop.
  People under 130 pounds should use one scoop, those 131–180 should use two scoops
  and those 181 and over should use three scoops.
† See Resources for recommended products and online sources for protein powders,
  leucine, and D-ribose.

SELECTING A PROTEIN POWDER

Back in the dark ages (1989), when *Thin So Fast* was published, we had to create a recipe for a meal-replacement protein powder because there simply was
none. Today, with the shelves of grocery and health food stores groaning under
the weight of all those protein powders on the market, it's hard to imagine
this. But except for a couple of really awful-tasting ones that only the hardest
of hard-core body builders could love (Joe Weider Milk and Egg Protein was
the best of the lot), these products didn't exist twenty years ago. Now they're
available everywhere—in stores, online, by direct mail. Your job is to select one
that you like the taste of that also meets the following criteria:

- It contains a minimum of 15 grams of protein per scoop (more is fine).
- It contains no more than 2 or 3 grams of carboydrate per scoop.
- It contains no aspartame sweetener. (Splenda, stevia, erythritol, xylitol, ri-
  bose, and acesulfame K are acceptable, if you tolerate them.)

Whey or whey protein isolates and egg are biologically the best proteins, but
if you are allergic to either, rice protein powder and soy protein powder are
acceptable substitutes as long as they do not contain significant additional carbohydrates.

cholesterol in the blood (if that itself even matters to health, which is
looking more and more doubtful) or to the increased risk of heart disease. Moreover, cholesterol is deeply important to human health, per-
forming a host of essential biochemical functions. Cholesterol serves as
a critical structural molecule in the membranes of every cell in the
body, as an important component of brain and nervous tissues, and as
the base molecule from which we make our gender-specific reproductive hormones and vitamin D, to name but a few of its jobs. Every cell in
the body can make cholesterol, though most cholesterol production
comes from the liver. The system operates on a feedback loop such that,

the more cholesterol we eat the less we must make, and the less cholesterol we eat, the more we must make. We don't need to eat *less* cholesterol; we need to eat *more,* even those of us trying to lower our blood
cholesterol and especially those of us trying to lose middle-body fat.

While most men are typically big red-meat eaters—one good source
of cholesterol—folks mistakenly concerned about its reputation for
driving up risk of heart disease (often women) eschew red meat and
eggs, preferring the white meat from chicken, fish, or seafood. If this
pattern describes your eating habits, we encourage you to add a single
raw egg (or just the yolk) to at least one shake a day. Even if you eat
cooked eggs, you may still want to supplement your shakes with an egg,
and here's why. The cholesterol in an egg yolk is easily oxidized in cooking; the longer you cook the egg, the higher the risk of oxidizing the
cholesterol in it, particularly in cooking methods involving breaking the
yolk, such as for scrambled eggs and omelets. Oxidized cholesterol (as
opposed to the nonoxidized kind) is more readily incorporated into
plaque in the arteries. Keeping the yolk intact during cooking and min-
imizing the cooking time to just long enough to solidify the white helps
preserve the quality of the cholesterol. By not cooking the egg at all,
however, you'll get the cholesterol in its purest and most beneficial
form.

Granted, there is a slight risk in consuming raw eggs, as they are potentially a source of salmonella bacteria and, thus, of food poisoning.
Fortunately, you can virtually eliminate this risk if you purchase eggs
that have been pasteurized in the shell. These eggs, available at most
grocery stores, are always labeled as having been pasteurized and usually each shell is stamped with a "P" in a circle on its end to indicate
pasteurization. If your store doesn't carry them, speak to the dairy man-
ager; they can get them from their supplier and will if there's a market
for them. If you cannot find pasteurized eggs, you can add some measure of safety to standard raw eggs simply by giving them a 30- to 60-
second dunk (whole in the shell) in boiling water. Don't leave them too
long or you'll cook the whites. After their swim in the hot tub, remove

them, cool them under cold running water, mark them with your own "P," and store them in the refrigerator to use within a few days.

Although adding an egg to your Power Up! Protein Shake will help boost middle-body fat loss, we recommend you do so only when you make the shake fresh and drink it right away. If you will be eating on the run and need to take the shake in a thermos, for instance, or make it ahead and put it into the refrigerator to drink later, omit the egg— even a pasteurized one—as an added measure of food safety.

POWER UP! SHAKE FLAVORINGS

In working with thousands and thousands of patients on this dietary regimen, we found that some people are devoted to a single flavor, content to have the same pure and simple chocolate,* vanilla, or straw-berry shake time and again. If that describes you, your job is an easy one: just pick the flavor of protein powder you love and follow the basic shake recipe. If variety is what you crave, however, you'll want to have a number of ingredients on hand to be able to whip up just the taste you're looking for at a moment's notice. Begin by choosing a suitable protein powder that is available in all three basic flavors— vanilla, chocolate, and strawberry. Then make a dash to the spice aisle of your grocery store to pick up a variety of extracts, as used in the recipes. (Check out the Resources for online sources of other interest-ing flavor extracts.) You may also want to pick up some sugar-free cof-fee syrups (from Torini or DaVinci) to add even more depth to your flavor chart.

Once you've got your flavoring pantry well stocked, you can begin mak-ing your shakes. To the basic Power Up! ProteinShake recipe (page 115), make the additions or substitutions specified in the Flavor Variations

---

* We know—we said no caffeine. While pure cocoa does have some theobromine in it (a rel-ative of caffeine), the amount used to flavor shake powder shouldn't give you enough to matter. If you feel it does affect you, opt for other flavor choices.

that follow to create a mouth-watering array of options. With this many choices—you can pick a different one for every day, if you like—you'll never get bored.

Wild Berry Substitute half the ice with ½ cup frozen unsweetened mixed berries; use strawberry-flavored protein powder.

Caramel Cappuccino Use vanilla protein powder; substitute 1 cup of cold decaf coffee for the water, and add 1 to 2 tablespoons of Torino or DaVinci sugar-free caramel syrup.

Turtle Sundae Use chocolate protein powder; add 1 tablespoon each of Torino or DaVinci sugar-free caramel syrup and sugar-free hazelnut syrup.

White Chocolate Mocha Café Use chocolate protein powder; substitute 1 cup cold decaf coffee for the water and add 1 to 2 tablespoons of Torini or DaVinci sugar-free white chocolate syrup.

Black Forest Cake Use chocolate protein powder; substitute 6 ounces of diet black cherry soda for the water. (See important sidebar on making shakes with sodas, page 121.)

Orange Sherbet Use vanilla protein powder; substitute 6 ounces of diet orange soda for the water; add 1 teaspoon fresh grated orange zest, if desired. (See important sidebar on making shakes with sodas, page 121.)

Piña Colada Use vanilla protein powder; substitute 1 ounce of premium coconut milk for the heavy cream; add ½ teaspoon each of pineapple extract, coconut extract, and rum flavoring.

Bananas Foster Use vanilla protein powder; add 1 teaspoon banana extract and 1 tablespoon Torino or DaVinci sugar-free caramel syrup.

Coconut Cream Pie Use vanilla protein powder; substitute ¼ cup premium coconut milk for ¼ cup of the water, but do not omit the heavy cream; add ½ teaspoon coconut extract and 1 tablespoon sugar-free Torini or DaVinci hazelnut syrup.

Peaches and Cream Use vanilla protein powder; substitute 6 ounces diet Hansen's Peach soda for the water. (See important sidebar about making shakes with sodas, page 121.)

Strawberry Sundae Use strawberry protein powder; substitute 1 cup frozen unsweetened strawberries for the ice; top with an added dollop of whipped cream, sweetened artificially with Splenda, stevia, xylitol, or erythritol to make it especially rich, if desired.

Peppermint Patty Use chocolate protein powder; add 1 tablespoon Torini or DaVinci sugar-free chocolate syrup and ½ teaspoon mint extract.

Rum Runner Punch Use strawberry protein powder; for water, substitute 6 ounces diet tangerine and lime soda and add ½ teaspoon each pineapple extract and rum extract. (See important sidebar about making shakes with sodas, page 121.)

Egg Nog Use vanilla protein powder; add 1 teaspoon rum extract and a pinch of freshly grated nutmeg.

Chai Latte Use vanilla protein powder; replace ½ cup of the water with ½ cup Sugar-Free Oregon Chai.

THE PRESCRIBED MEALS

Every day during Weeks 1 and 2, choose one of the prescribed meals as your solid meal of the day. You'll notice that many of the dishes in the menus are marked with an asterisk (*). This symbol denotes that the full recipe for that dish appears in the Recipe section of the book. We've

MAKING SHAKES WITH SODAS

Diet sodas made with Splenda come in an ever-widening variety of flavors that make great substitutes for the plain water in the basic shake recipe. One important caveat in making shakes using sodas, however, is that their carbonation can cause them to erupt in the blender if not carefully handled. One option is to first open the container and let the beverage go flat, losing its fizz. But if that doesn't appeal and you are using a fresh can or bottle of diet soda, place your hand firmly over the lid of the blender jar and hold it tightly while blending the shake or you could find your breakfast all over your counter ... or your ceiling.

grouped the menus into categories—breakfast, lunch, dinner—and have designed the meals to offer enough options to keep your yearning for variety appeased.

You may enjoy your meal at any time of day that is convenient, selecting from the breakfast, lunch, or dinner menus that follow. Feel free to omit any of the meals you do not like, to repeat any meals that you enjoy, or to try them all. But remember: *for the first two weeks, eat only one meal per day.* Don't worry that you will be hungry; your delicious meal will be in addition to three filling Power Up! Protein Shakes each day, and we assure you that you will be well fed at the cellular level. In very short order—usually within a day or two—your metabolism will respond to this structure for eating and you will feel neither deprived nor hungry—just energized and already leaner.

TAILORING THE MEALS

You will notice that we have not specified the amounts of most protein foods—meats, fish, poultry, eggs, seafood—in the menus that follow, but we have routinely specified portions for the fruits, vegetables, some dairy, starchier foods, and breads. That's because we want you to eat the amount of protein that satisfies your hunger. Bigger bodies and bigger appetites generally need 6 to 8 ounces of protein, small bodies and appetites generally require 3 to 4 ounces, and middle-size ones want something in between. But those are just general guidelines. While we don't want you to stuff yourself, whatever your size, we want you to eat a generous enough portion of protein to feel full; after all, it's your only solid meal of the day and protein is critical to successful weight loss. All the basic protein choices are interchangeable, as well. If you love beef but don't care for lamb, substitute beef for lamb in a given menu; if you're not a fish eater, substitute poultry or meat for the fish or seafood. The point is to get enough good-quality protein at your meal.

During this two-week period, however, we do want you to limit your carbohydrate intake to achieve one important goal: reducing insulin and blood sugar levels, which will boost fat burning, discourage fat storage, and speed the removal of fat from the liver cells. We've provided you with a wide selection of fruits and vegetables that are tasty and packed with micronutrients but low in available starch and sugar. Within a given meal, we've combined fruits, vegetables, and (occasional) breads in particular amounts, designed to provide a prescribed total amount of carbohydrate. But if there is an item on the menu that you can't or won't eat, modify the menu by substituting another item. To keep the total carbohydrate content of your meals within acceptable limits for Weeks 1 and 2, check the Food Substitutions Lists for fruits and vegetables (Appendix) to find suitable alternatives to the item you don't like or can't eat. Now all you have to do is start eating!

Prescribed Breakfast Choices

1. Confetti Omelet* with crisp bacon (or turkey bacon)
   3 tomato slices, sprinkled with Celtic Sea Salt
   Water, mineral water, white or herbal tea, or decaf coffee or tea

---

* Recipe can be found in the Recipe section of this book.

2. Asparagus and Bacon Crustless Quiche*

    ½ cup fresh or unsweetened frozen strawberries (sweetened
        with a sprinkle of Splenda, xylitol, erythritol, or stevia, if
        desired)

    Water, mineral water, white or herbal tea, or decaf coffee or tea

3. Egg and Sausage Pie*

    ½ cup mixed berries

    Water, mineral water, white or herbal tea, or decaf coffee or tea

4. Goldilox Scramble*

    ½ cup cherry tomato halves, with a sprinkling of capers and
        diced red onion (drizzled with olive oil vinaigrette, or your
        choice of dressing, if desired)

    ½ cup fresh melon cubes with a squeeze of fresh lime juice and
        grated lime zest

    Water, mineral water, white or herbal tea, or decaf coffee or tea

5. Florentine Scramble*

    ½ cup fresh raspberries

    Water, mineral water, white or herbal tea, or decaf coffee
        or tea

6. 2 or 3 Lemon Ricotta Flapjacks*

    Crisp bacon (turkey or pork)

    ½ cup fresh blackberries

    Water, decaf coffee, decaf or herbal tea

7. 1 Powered-up Waffle* with melted butter and Sugar-Free Maple
        Syrup*

    2 or 3 sausage links (turkey or pork)

    2 or 3 fresh orange slices

    Water, decaf coffee, decaf or herbal tea

8. Hard-boiled eggs

    Smoked salmon slices

    3 or 4 fresh tomato slices, with a sprinkling of diced red onion
        and capers

    Water, mineral water, white or herbal tea, or decaf coffee or tea

9. Poached Eggs on Herbed Broiled Tomato Slices*
    Sausage patties or crisp bacon (pork or turkey)
    ½ cup sautéed spinach
    ½ cup fresh melon
    Water, mineral water, white or herbal tea, or decaf coffee or tea
10. Powered-up Kefir and Fresh Berries*
    Crisp bacon or sausage patties (pork or turkey)
    Water, mineral water, white or herbal tea, or decaf coffee or tea

Prescribed Lunch Choices

1. Chicken Caesar Salad Lettuce Wraps*
    ½ cup grapes
    Water, mineral water, white or herbal tea, or decaf coffee or tea
2. Broiled lamb (or beef) burger, "protein-style"†
    1 cup Mediterranean Chopped Salad*
    2 slices Grilled Haloumi*
    Water, mineral water, white or herbal tea, or decaf coffee
        or tea
3. 1½ cups Very Chickeny (or Beefy) Vegetable Soup*
    1 small low-carb flour tortilla, buttered
    1 small green salad with olive oil vinaigrette
    Water, mineral water, white or herbal tea, or decaf coffee or tea
4. 1 or 2 bunless chili-cheese dogs
    1 cup Crunchy Cabbage Slaw*
    ½ small apple
    Water, mineral water, white or herbal tea, or decaf coffee
        or tea

---

† "Protein-style" in reference to sandwiches and burgers means ditching the buns and wrapping the insides in a couple of large crunchy lettuce leaves instead. Big iceberg lettuce leaves work well for this purpose, but large leaves of romaine, green leaf, red leaf, or Boston Bibb lettuce work as well. Many restaurants have jumped on the idea and offer their burgers and chicken sandwiches in this manner.

5. BLAT Lettuce Wrap*

   2 to 3 ounces brie cheese

   ½ cup grapes

   Water, mineral water, white or herbal tea, or decaf coffee
   or tea

6. Chef's salad (lettuce, ¼ cup grated carrot, ¼ cup diced tomato,
   hard-boiled egg with choice of diced ham, turkey, or chicken
   and crumbled bacon, if desired; grated Cheddar or crumbled
   feta or blue cheese), and ranch, blue cheese, or olive oil
   vinaigrette dressing

   Water, mineral water, white or herbal tea, or decaf coffee
   or tea

7. Buffalo Chicken Wings*

   Salad of mixed greens dressed with blue cheese dressing, or
   dressing of choice†

   ½ cup each carrot and celery sticks

   Water, mineral water, white or herbal tea, or decaf or tea.

8. Chicken (or Tuna) Salad Stuffed Tomato,* with olive oil
   vinaigrette or dressing of choice

   ½ small apple

   1 or 2 ounces Cheddar or Monterey jack cheese

   Water, mineral water, white or herbal tea, or decaf coffee or tea

9. Classic Cobb Salad* with blue cheese dressing or dressing of
   choice

   4 to 5 Blue Diamond Almond Nut Thin crackers with butter

   ½ cup grapes for dessert

   Water, mineral water, white or herbal tea, or decaf coffee or tea

10. Grilled chicken breast, "protein-style," dressed with your choice
    mayo, mustard, pickle, and ketchup

    1 small orange or tangerine

    Water, mineral water, white or herbal tea, or decaf coffee or tea

† Any dressing used should contain fewer than 3 grams of carbohydrate per serving.

Prescribed Dinner Choices

1.   Herb-Roasted Chicken*

    4 or 5 baby carrots, steamed, with butter, salt, and pepper

    ½ cup Broccoli Amondine*

    ½ cup fresh or frozen raspberries topped with a dollop of Sweet Lime Cream*

    Water, mineral water, white or herbal tea, or decaf coffee or tea

2.   Grilled Spice-Rubbed Flank Steak*

    2 cups fresh spinach, sautéed in olive oil with minced garlic

    1 medium tomato, sliced, salted, and drizzled with olive oil and balsamic vinegar

    ½ cup fresh or frozen blackberries, topped with 1 to 2 tablespoons heavy cream

    Water, mineral water, white or herbal tea, or decaf coffee or tea

3.   Grilled Citrus-Rosemary Salmon*

    ½ cup Creamy Cauliflower Puree*

    ½ recipe Broiled Herbed Tomato Halves*

    1 cup fresh mixed lettuces, dressed with balsamic vinaigrette

    ½ fresh peach, sliced, topped with a dollop of Sweet Lime Cream*

    Water, mineral water, white or herbal tea, or decaf coffee or tea

4.   Garlic-Rubbed Pork Tenderloin*

    ½ cup Sautéed Apples and Red Cabbage*

    5 or 6 spears roasted or steamed asparagus with olive oil, salt, and pepper

    ½ cup Strawberry, Mandarin, and Mint Cup*

    Water, mineral water, white or herbal tea, or decaf coffee or tea

5.   Rosemary and Mint Lamb Chops*

    1 cup Mediterranean Chopped Salad*

    2 slices Grilled Haloumi*

    Water, mineral water, white or herbal tea, or decaf coffee or tea

6.   Triple Threat Meatloaf *

    ½ cup Creamy Cauliflower Puree*

½ cup seasoned steamed green beans

1 serving Savory Sautéed Apple Slices*

Water, mineral water, white or herbal tea or decaf coffee or tea

7. Lamb and Red Pepper Kebab* on a bed of Herbed Cauli-Rice*

   1 cup Greek Salad* with ⅛ cup Minted Yogurt Dressing*

   ½ Grilled Plum* with a splash of balsamic vinegar

   Water, mineral water, white or herbal tea, or decaf coffee
      or tea

8. Grilled steak

   5 or 6 spears roasted asparagus, sprinkled with salt and drizzled
      with olive oil

   ½ cup Creamy Cauliflower Puree*

   4 or 5 steamed baby carrots, sprinkled with olive oil, rosemary,
      and sea salt

   ½ cup fresh strawberries, with whipped cream, if desired

   Water, mineral water, white or herbal tea, or decaf coffee or tea

9. San-J Traditional White Miso Soup† (optional)

   Thai Chicken Lettuce Wraps*

   Fried Cauli-Rice*

   Water, mineral water, white or herbal tea, or decaf coffee or tea

10. Pork Tenderloin Roast*

   ½ cup Creamy Cauliflower Puree*

   1 (canned) roasted red pepper, seasoned with olive oil, salt, and
      pepper

   1 serving Savory Sautéed Apple Slices*

   Water, mineral water, decaf coffee, decaf or herbal tea

11. Stuffed Buffalo (or Beef) Burgers*

   Sunny Day Garden Salad* with dressing of your choice

   ½ cup fresh raspberries with a dollop of whipped cream

   Water, mineral water, white or herbal tea, or decaf coffee or tea

---

† San J Traditional White Miso Soup is a commercial dry mix, prepared by simply adding hot water.

12. Lemon Chicken*

    ½ cup zucchini sautéed in butter with garlic, salt, and pepper

    3 or 4 tomato slices sprinkled with sea salt and a drizzle of
        olive oil

    ½ cup diced fresh melon

    Water, mineral water, white or herbal tea, or decaf coffee or tea

13. Speedy Garlic Shrimp*

    ½ cup steamed spaghetti squash tossed with olive oil, salt, and
        pepper

    ½ cup Parmesan Broccoli and Red Peppers*

    Water, mineral water, white or herbal tea, or decaf coffee or tea

14. Fish and Peppers Packets*

    ½ cup mushrooms, sautéed in olive oil, garlic, and thyme

    ½ Grilled Nectarine* with a dollop of whipped cream, if desired

    Water, mineral water, white or herbal tea, or decaf coffee or tea

ASSESSING YOUR PROGRESS

At the end of Week 2 of The Cure, repeat your measurements and
weight, and jot them down on your Initial Assessment and Progress
Log (page 285). Now you're ready to move on to the next chapter, where
you'll learn what to do in Weeks 3 and 4, and get to enjoy even more delicious food on your way to curing the curse of the middle-aged middle.
Before you move on, however, don't forget to give blood.

7

THE CURE: WEEKS 3 AND 4
(THE MEAT WEEKS)

"Wish I had time for just one more bowl of chili."
—Kit Carson's last words

After two weeks of the calorie-controlled, prescribed food intake necessary to reset your metabolic balance, drop your insulin levels, and purge the liver cells of much of their fat, you're now ready to move into the next phase of The Cure. In Weeks 3 and 4, you'll raise the caloric stakes by eating more protein, and especially more fats, while even more sharply controlling the carbohydrate portion of your diet. The purpose of this dietary structural change is threefold: to provide plenty of calories to preserve your metabolic drive, to supply plenty of protein to preserve your lean tissues (your muscles, bone, hair, skin, nails, blood, brain, heart, and other vital organs), and to offer very few carbohydrates to ensure that your insulin level stays low, thus blunting the fat-storage signals your body receives as you increase your caloric intake.

Fat storage is driven in two ways by diet: hormonally and by an excess of calories. By "hormonally," in this case, we're not referring to the

drop in gender-specific reproductive hormone levels (estrogen, progesterone, and testosterone) or the regulatory hormones (thyroid), described in Chapter 2, that can alter body shape, muscularity, and fat
storage. Rather we mean the hormones of glucose (blood sugar) metabolism, and chiefly the impact of elevated levels of the hormone insulin
and its opposite, glucagon.

Unlike levels of the reproductive hormones, we can almost completely influence—for better or worse—the levels of these metabolic
hormones by what we eat. How our food choices impact the metabolic
hormones concerns not so much the number of calories we consume,
but their quality—that is, are they coming from protein, carbs, or fat?
Although it may seem trivial, it most assuredly is not and here's why.

All calories are not created equal. The metabolic impact of protein is
balanced, raising the blood levels of both the fat-storage hormone, insulin, and the fat-mobilizing hormone, glucagon. The rise in insulin
occasioned by eating protein is necessary to drive the amino-acid building blocks (into which dietary proteins are deconstructed by digestion)
into the cells, so that the body can use them to build and maintain muscle and other lean tissues. The rise in glucagon transmits two equally
important messages to the body: to make a slow, steady supply of blood
sugar from some of the incoming protein and to unload the fat stores
and burn their contents for energy. The rise in protein intake during
Weeks 3 and 4 assures your body of having plenty of the amino-acid raw
materials it will need to preserve lean tissues and to make blood sugar
while your carb intake is low.

The metabolic impact of carbohydrate (whether complex or simple,
starch or sugar) serves to sharply raise the output of insulin without the
balancing effect of glucagon. This imbalance signals to the body to
store fat—preferentially in the middle—and as a result deprives the
cells of a reliable fuel source from which to make the energy they need
to survive. Cellular energy starvation is a powerful stimulus to appetite
because it prompts the cells to send out an SOS that triggers the release
of a firestorm of hormones and neurotransmitters (body chemicals that

transmit specific messages to the cells), designed to raise blood sugar as an emergency fuel source. The result is hunger and carbohydrate craving.

The effect of fat on the metabolic hormones, on the other hand, is quite neutral, causing no rise in either of these important regulators. Good-quality fat serves simply as high-octane fuel when your body is in metabolic balance. When the hormonal signals are working properly, as they should be after your introductory two weeks, the cells of the body will burn fat as their preferred fuel to make energy for doing the myriad jobs a body must do minute by minute, day in and day out. Having a plentiful supply of the right kind of calories (both from what you eat and from opening the spigot of your own middle-body fat stores) acts to prevent hunger and the cellular energy starvation that comes from a diet too low in calories, too low in fat, too low in protein, and too high in carbohydrate.

The design of Weeks 3 and 4 of The Cure, therefore, relies mainly on the single best source of high-quality protein and fat: meat. In the meal plans that follow, you'll enjoy "meat" in all its forms: beef, pork, lamb, poultry, fish, seafood, game, and eggs. If you are a vegetarian, these two weeks of meals are obviously not ideal for you. But if you are willing to consume eggs and/or fish or poultry, the section at the end of the chapter has some instructions on how to approximate the effect of an essentially all-meat diet without eating meat. If you are a committed vegan, the unfortunate reality is that it's nearly impossible to adopt this structure and keep your carbohydrate intake low enough to make a substantial metabolic correction and still get enough nonanimal protein. It's very tough, and pretty boring, to do it using soy-based proteins alone, albeit even for just two weeks.

THE RULES OF THE GAME—WEEKS 3 AND 4

1. You may reintroduce alcohol, in limited quantity, during this phase of the plan. Twice a week, your choice of when, you can enjoy a single

4-ounce glass of dry red or white wine, or a single 12-ounce light beer, or a single shot (about 1½ ounces) of distilled spirits. One drink, twice a week. We can attest (from our own experience and that with countless patients) that it's very easy to slip back into a pattern of drinking more and more often. While there are benefits to moderate alcohol intake, weight loss is not one of them. When you drink too much alcohol, you slow the middle-body fat loss substantially; and since that's the name of this game, you must really work to avoid overdoing it until you have completed The Cure, or you will definitely undermine your progress. If you find that one drink leads to two, leads to three, you should probably put yourself back on the total alcohol prohibition of Weeks 1 and 2, in the interest of fat loss.

2. You may reintroduce caffeine, in moderate quantities. By that, we mean not more than two or three cups of caffeinated coffee per day. Contrary to coffee's somewhat bad reputation, scientific research suggests that a few cups of a caffeinated beverage (particularly coffee) may reduce your risk for Alzheimer's disease, Parkinson's disease, and diabetes. However, if you lighten your coffee or tea, limit your intake during these two weeks of the plan to a single lightened cup a day, with just a touch of half-and-half or cream; the balance of any coffee intake should be black. If you sweeten your coffee or tea, use a noncaloric sweetener, such as sucralose, stevia, or sugar alcohols.*

3. Eat meals of meat, fish, poultry, game, and eggs throughout the day in amounts sufficient to satisfy your appetite. We've designed the suggested meal plans for Weeks 3 and 4 as a guide and to demonstrate that a nearly all-meat diet can be quite varied. There is no specific restriction on the *amount* of meat that you should eat; just eat until you're full,

---

* We recommend that you avoid the use of aspartame (Equal) because research suggests that it may be harmful to the brain and nervous system and that the deleterious effect may be magnified on a lower carbohydrate diet.

then quit. When you get hungry, eat another meat meal or snack. On the lower end (and this will usually apply more to women than to men, since by and large men are bigger meat eaters anyway), be sure to eat at least three 3- to 4-ounce meat meals each day.

The meals should be fat-rich meals; no skinless boneless, steamed, or poached chicken or fish. Treat yourself to the skin; roast or sauté it in butter, olive oil, coconut oil, and herbs. And no bland steamed broccoli or asparagus; enjoy the butter, olive oil, sesame oil, and coconut oil that carry the flavor and serve as vehicles for the absorption of critical micronutrients. Try other healthy oils, such as walnut oil, avocado oil, macadamia nut oil, or Enova brand oil in vinaigrettes and marinades. The goal during this two-week stretch is to drive your metabolism upward by the availability of lots of high-octane fuel that can be burned, but that, with few carbohydrates and thus the absence of a strong insulin surge, won't be easily stored.

4. No dairy intake during these two weeks. Apart from a splash of cream in your cup of morning coffee or tea (and only if you must) and butter for cooking, as noted in Rule 3, you should avoid dairy products during Weeks 3 and 4. One of the pitfalls of attempts at continued weight loss, especially for women, is excessive consumption of cheese and cream. During this two-week interval in the plan you want to keep calories up but carbs quite low. Even though there aren't many carbs in cheese or cream—just a gram or two per serving—if the number of servings rises, the total can disrupt the steady loss of fat from the fat stores.

Additionally, these foods are dense in calories and easy to eat to excess. Over the years we've had many patients whose weight loss stalled when they ate more than tiny amounts of dairy products—for reasons that we cannot readily explain in metabolic or biochemical terms. We've heard it from enough people, though, that we believe it. For most people, although 1 tablespoon of cream in a cup of coffee probably won't do much, a tablespoon in each of 6 or 8 cups of coffee throughout the day does make an impact. (The same is true for nuts and nut butters. A tablespoon or two now and then won't hurt, but it's very easy for 1 tablespoon to become 8 tablespoons—and in the case of nut butters, for a couple grams of carb to become 20 grams.)

5. No grains or things made of them. Because grains are mainly just starch, and starch is just chains of sugar, these foods drive levels of blood sugar and insulin up and increase triglycerides, which as you've learned will fatten your middle. Avoid wheat, corn, rice, oats, barley, spelt, quinoa, amaranth, and other cereals, as well as their flours or meals during these two weeks of The Cure.

6. No starchy vegetables or legumes. That means no potatoes, no dried beans or peas, no foods made from them or their meals or flours.

7. You may resume taking the medications listed in the box on page 107, but only if necessary. Unlike alcohol and caffeine, both of which can put some degree of detoxification load on the liver but have clear health benefits when used properly, most medications aren't needed on a daily basis. We recommend taking over-the-counter and prescription medications, particularly those with a liver impact, as infrequently as is possible. Now that your liver is in better shape, let's keep it that way!

8. Continue to take your leucine. An additional 6 to 8 grams of leucine each day during Weeks 3 and 4 will help to preserve lean body tissues (muscle and bone) and to encourage middle-body fat loss. You can simply swallow the BCAA capsules, or you may prefer making them into a between-meal beverage we call muscle preserving drink (MPD). We make this ourselves by mixing about 2 grams of leucine powder (or an equivalent amount from the contents of BCAA capsules), plus 1 single-serving packet of Lipton's Sugar Free Green Tea to Go, with 8 to 10 ounces of water in a refillable water bottle. The amino acids are a tad sour or even bitter, and somewhat insoluble in cold water, but keep shaking and they'll finally mostly dissolve. If you're aiming for 6 to 8 grams a day, then drink three or four of these MPDs per day and you'll be there.

9. Continue to take your vitamins. As far as added vitamins and minerals go, a supplement that provides at least the RDI of all nutrients is all that is absolutely necessary this week and the next; just an over-the-counter recommended minimum-daily-requirement multivitamin/mineral will do. We still recommend taking some added potassium and magnesium during these two weeks, since your carbohydrate intake will remain low and consequently you may still waste some potassium. If you aren't a good supplement taker, this minimum recommendation will be music to your ears. Many people, however, are both believers in the benefits of larger dose supplementation and feel comfortable taking supplemental nutrients. Others perhaps have specific health goals whereby taking supplements beyond the basics can prove valuable. Rest assured; it's quite all right to continue the full-supplement regimen from Weeks 1 and 2, if you so desire; the full regimen is actually quite good for you—it's just not critical to your success on the plan. (See Resources for online sources for supplements.)

10. Continue to hydrate yourself well. Since you're still in the fat-burning mode, you'll want to drink plenty of water to support that work, and with insulin levels low, you won't retain it as you would on a high-carb diet. The source could be water or any water-based, carb- and calorie-free beverage (again, preferably not sweetened with aspartame).

11. If you feel hungry, eat more fat and protein. Try a small burger patty, a few slices of smoked salmon, hard-boiled or deviled eggs, left-over steak or chicken, or even a tablespoonful of olive oil—but do not eat bigger servings of vegetables. The vegetables chosen for this week, in the quantities suggested, should provide no more than 5 or 6 effective (net) grams of carbohydrate per meal. In order to achieve the

> ## TO YOUR HEALTH
>
> Moderate consumption of alcohol—defined as a drink or two a day, not every day—has been associated in many studies with a lowered risk of cardiovascular diseases, a reduction in blood pressure, an elevation in HDL (the so-called good cholesterol) and, surprisingly, improved weight loss over that of strict teetotalers. Remember, too, that wine and beer have a carb cost you'll need to consider. Dry wines contain about a gram of carbohydrate per ounce; a light beer, about 3 to 5 grams per 12-ounce serving. Therefore, even though a little is good, don't get carried away with it. Alcohol in greater quantities has just the opposite effect and can wreak havoc with the liver, leading to fatty infiltration of the liver and storage of middle-body fat. Regarding the use of alcohol, the ancient Greeks said it best: strive for moderation in all things.

metabolic goals you're after, it is imperative that this two-week stretch be one higher in calories, but very, very low in carbohydrates.

A VARIED, NEARLY ALL-MEAT DIET

If you consider yourself a big meat eater, you may be jumping for joy at the idea of a meat diet, thinking "What could be easier or tastier?" Others of you may be thinking, "Meat? Just meat?" If you're cringing as you imagine two long weeks of eating nothing but meat, relax! "Meat," in our parlance, is a much broader category than you might imagine. As you'll see when you look at the suggested meal plans that follow, our varied, nearly all-meat diet, in addition to the typical beef, lamb, pork, and game, includes poultry, eggs, fish, seafood, and even a selection of specific vegetables chosen for their high-nutrient density at a very low-carb cost. No matter your meat-eating affinity, short of those subscribing to a strict vegan ideology, you're sure to find something to love and you'll be surprised at how easy and satisfying these two weeks will be.

Make the design of these two weeks work for you. Remember that the meal plans are simply our suggestions of what you might eat. As was the case in Weeks 1 and 2, if you see an item in a breakfast, lunch, or dinner you don't like or can't eat, simply substitute a different green vegetable or dark leafy green from the Meat Week Fruit and Vegetable Substitutions Lists (see Appendix) for it. If you're happy eating the same thing—be it steak, salmon, or chicken—five nights a week, go for it! Also, as before, the meal suggestions don't specify an amount of the eggs, meat, fish, poultry, seafood, or game, but they do specify *exact amounts* of what goes with it—the fruit or vegetable portion of the meal. Eat enough of the protein (meat) portion to satisfy your hunger, but don't overdo it. Typical portions are 6 to 8 ounces for big people and big appetites, 3 to 4 ounces for small people and small appetites, and something in between for people mid-range in appetite and body size. And limit your intake of the fruits and vegetables to no more than what's listed in the Meat Weeks meal plans or the substitution guidelines.

We designed the meal plans (and recipes that accompany them) for people who cook—they're recipes, after all, which implies cooking. You'll notice that we've also given some "Meat Week Variations" to some of the recipes that you used in Weeks 1 and 2, adjusted to eliminate dairy and any other ingredient off-limits during Weeks 3 and 4. The great majority of recipes are quick and simple to prepare, and they're all delicious. But what if you don't cook, or don't have the time to do so every night? We've got you covered, too, with "Take-out and Restaurant Substitutions" and a selection of quick and easy recipe tips that will teach you how to leverage your time in the kitchen. Armed with a little know-how, you can cook once and eat well for days.

COOK ONCE, EAT TWICE . . . OR THRICE

In this fast-paced world in which we juggle work, family, and friends, it's become increasingly hard to find the time to prepare meals at home. It's tough sometimes to even sit down to eat a nutritious dinner, let

A MEAT WEEK SHAKE OPTION

Although during these next two weeks your intake of dairy products is limited, if you get into a bind and simply don't have time for a meat meal, you may still occasionally have a protein shake—somewhat modified—in place of one meat meal. Simply use the premium coconut milk option in place of the heavy cream, as written in the Power Up! Protein Shake recipe (page 115). And remember that if you get into a really tight spot, just whipping up a shake with nothing but cold water and flavored protein powder is better than not eating enough protein or eating the wrong things.

alone find the time to cook a good meal every night and stick to your plan. The obligations of work, a social life, and volunteer responsibilities gobble up huge blocks of time and relegate meals to catch-as-catch-can. Add to that the responsibility of parents to shuttle kids or grandkids from soccer to ballet to children's choir to scouts, and it's easy to see why the family dinner has become nearly extinct. Sure, you can run through the fast-food line, grab a burger, ditch the bun, and eat on the fly—but where's the joy in that? With a little planning, you can manage to have your steak and eat it, too.

One easy way to do this is to leverage your kitchen time by making double or even triple batches of dishes that will freeze well or keep for several days in the refrigerator, and that will reheat quickly in the microwave or on the stovetop. One day's dinner can become the next day's lunch or dinner, and often with some minor modifications, it can be the lunch or dinner after that.

For instance, when you cook a chicken, it takes essentially no longer and no more energy to cook two chickens than one. You'll have the first as a roasted chicken for that night's dinner and the second as roast chicken again a night or two later, with a quick reheating, or to make it into chicken salad for lunches for a day or two, or into chicken soup for lunch or dinner the next day. During Weeks 3 and 4, the Meat Weeks, make a double or triple recipe of burgers—full-size patties for future meals and smaller (about 2-inch) patties for any time you need a quick snack. Make a double pot of chili or meaty soup to enjoy for multiple meals. Make a double batch of veggie side dishes, since most of them will reheat in a flash and still be delicious.

With that plan in mind, flip through the recipes in this book; you'll see that many have a "Time-saving Tip" at the end. These tips describe how to leverage one afternoon or evening's labor in the kitchen into several days' worth of meals.

Here are the suggested meal plans for Weeks 3 and 4—the Meat Weeks.

Suggested Breakfasts

1. Sausage, Egg, and Cheese Scramble* (Meat Weeks Variation)
    1 cup fresh spinach, sautéed with butter and garlic
    Water, mineral water, coffee, or tea

2. Ham and Asparagus Scramble*
    ½ medium tomato, sliced, salted, and drizzled with olive oil
    Water, mineral water, coffee, or tea

3. Poached Eggs on Herbed Broiled Tomato Slices*
    Crisp bacon (or turkey bacon) slices
    Water, mineral water, coffee, or tea

4. Hard-boiled eggs and smoked salmon slices
    ½ fresh tomato, sliced, salted, and drizzled with olive oil
    Water, mineral water, coffee, or tea

5. Confetti Omelet*
    Canadian bacon, ham, or turkey ham
    Water, mineral water, coffee, or tea

6. Deviled Eggs with Lox and Capers*
    ½ avocado, salted, drizzled with balsamic vinaigrette
    Water, mineral water, coffee, or tea

* Recipe can be found in the Recipe section of this book.

7.   Scrambled Egg Roll-Up*
     4 or 5 grapes (about ¼ cup)
     Water, mineral water, coffee, or tea
8.   Florentine Scramble*
     3 or 4 asparagus spears, cut in pieces, sautéed in butter
     Water, mineral water, coffee, or tea
9.   Eggs, fried in butter
     Crisp bacon
     ½ cup cherry tomato halves, salted lightly, tossed with olive oil
     Water, mineral water, coffee, or tea

Suggested Lunches

1.   Hamburger pattie(s), protein-style, between two crunchy lettuce
        leaves
     1 or 2 strips crisp bacon or turkey bacon
     ½ Hass avocado, sliced
     1 slice ripe tomato
     Mayo, mustard, dill pickle, as desired
     Water, mineral water, aspartame-free diet soda, coffee, or tea
2.   Naked chili dog(s) (no buns, no beans)
     Dill pickle relish, mustard, onions, as desired
     ½ cup Crunchy Cabbage Slaw*
     Water, mineral water, aspartame-free diet soda, coffee, or tea
3.   Rotisserie chicken (take-out or home-roasted)
     ½ cup Sunny Day Garden Salad*
     Water, mineral water, aspartame-free diet soda, coffee, or tea
4.   Meat Week Soup*
     1 to 2 cups green salad with Dijon Vinaigrette,* or choice of
        olive oil dressing
     Water, mineral water, aspartame-free diet soda, coffee, or tea
5.   Gyro Burger(s),* wrapped in crunchy lettuce leaves
     ½ cup Mediterranean Chopped Salad*
     Water, mineral water, aspartame-free diet soda, coffee, or tea

BREAKFAST TAKE-OUT AND RESTAURANT SUBSTITUTIONS

No matter where you are, you can always find a suitable breakfast. Just order eggs any style and/or your choice of sausage, bacon, ham, or smoked fish. Hold the bread.

If desired, and if they're available, you may also have any **one** of the following:

- ½ cup sautéed spinach or dark greens
- 1–2 slices of a medium tomato
- ½ avocado
- 3–4 asparagus spears
- ¼ cup of fresh berries
- 1 slice (¹⁄₁₆) of a small cantaloupe
- 1 slice of an orange
- 4–5 grapes

6. Chicken Caesar Salad Lettuce Wrap(s)*
   3 or 4 large strawberries
   Water, mineral water, aspartame-free diet soda, coffee, or tea
7. Antipasto Lunch Plate*
   Water, mineral water, aspartame-free diet soda, coffee, or tea
8. Inside Out Triple-Decker Ham Sandwich(es)*
   ½ cup Crunchy Cabbage Slaw*
   1 or 2 dill pickle spears
   Water, mineral water, aspartame-free diet soda, coffee, or tea
9. Gourmet Nutty Bird Burger(s),* protein-style, wrapped in
      crunchy lettuce leaves
   ¼ cup Cranberry-Orange Relish*
   1 or 2 dill pickle spears
   Water, mineral water, aspartame-free diet soda, coffee,
      or tea

> ## LUNCH AND DINNER TAKE-OUT
> ## AND RESTAURANT SUBSTITUTIONS
>
> - Roasted or grilled chicken or turkey piece(s) of your choice (prepared without breading), with green salad, oil and vinegar dressing, or ½ cup any green vegetable (green beans, broccoli, asparagus, cauliflower, cabbage, spinach, or other dark greens). Ask for melted butter for your vegetables, if available, or drizzle them with a little olive oil.
> - Double bacon burger, no bun, add avocado if available, one slice of tomato, with green salad and oil and vinegar dressing.
> - Grilled or broiled salmon (or other fish or shellfish prepared without breading), with green salad and ½ cup any green vegetable. Ask for melted butter for your fish and/or vegetables, if available, or again, drizzle them with olive oil.
> - Steak, green salad, and ½ cup green vegetable. Ask for melted butter for your vegetables, if available, or drizzle on some olive oil.
> - Sashimi (any type fish or shellfish), green or cucumber salad, no rice. Select fatty fish (fatty tuna, salmon, mackerel) if available.

10. Thai Chicken Lettuce Wraps*
    1 or 2 dill pickle spears or ¼ cup pepperoncini rings
    Water, mineral water, aspartame-free diet soda, coffee, or tea

Suggested Dinners

1. Grilled Citrus-Rosemary Salmon*
   4 or 5 roasted asparagus spears, with butter, salt, and pepper
   Water, mineral water, aspartame-free diet soda, coffee,
      or tea
2. Lamb and Red Pepper Kebabs*
   1 cup salad greens with olive oil vinaigrette
   Water, mineral water, aspartame-free diet soda, coffee, or tea

3. Grilled Spice-Rubbed Flank Steak*
    ½ cup seasoned green beans, with butter, garlic, salt, and pepper
    ¼ medium tomato, in wedges, with olive oil vinaigrette
    Water, mineral water, aspartame-free diet soda, coffee, or tea

4. Chicken with 40 Cloves of Garlic*
    ½ cup Herbed Cauli-Rice*
    1 cup salad greens, with olive oil vinaigrette
    Water, mineral water, aspartame-free diet soda, coffee, or tea

5. Fish and Peppers Packets*
    1 cup salad greens, with olive oil vinaigrette
    Water, mineral water, aspartame-free diet soda, coffee, or tea

6. Speedy Garlic Shrimp*
    2 cups Warm Sesame and Ginger Spinach Salad*
    ½ Hass avocado, sliced, sprinkled with lemon juice, salt, and
        pepper
    Water, mineral water, aspartame-free diet soda, coffee, or tea.

7. Triple-Threat Meatloaf*
    ½ cup green beans, seasoned with butter, salt, and pepper
    ½ cup Creamy Cauliflower Puree*
    Water, mineral water, aspartame-free diet soda, coffee, or tea

8. Grilled steak with green salad and olive oil dressing
    1 serving Parmesan Broccoli and Red Peppers* (Meat Week
        Variation)
    Water, mineral water, aspartame-free diet soda, coffee, or tea

9. Garlic-Rubbed Pork Tenderloin*
    ½ cup Sautéed Apples and Red Cabbage* (Meat Week Variation)
    ¼ cup Olive Salad*
    Water, mineral water, aspartame-free diet soda, coffee, or tea

10. Lemon Chicken*
    ½ cup Herbed Cauli-Rice*
    ½ cup sautéed fresh spinach, with garlic, olive oil, salt, and
        pepper
    Water, mineral water, aspartame-free diet soda, coffee, or tea

Keep up your salt intake. Odd as it may seem to hear a doctor tell you to eat salt, when you're following a meat diet that contains virtually no starch or sugar, you may need to do just that. Enjoy a cup of salty bouillon, a dill pickle spear, a bit of dill pickle juice, or a few olives once or twice a day, and salt your food a bit more with sea salt to keep your sodium intake up. If you feel light-headed or slightly woozy when you stoop and stand, then you need more sodium.

FOR VEGETARIANS ONLY

An all-meat diet presents a challenge to those who subscribe to a vegetarian way of life, but not an insurmountable one. The goal is to provide plenty of protein and good fats and not many carb grams. Those ends can be met with some fairly minor adjustments and substitutions to the meal plans and recipes.

You will be able to pretty easily modify the breakfast options, simply by omitting the bacon, sausage, or ham in any recipe or replacing it with baked tofu, smoked fish, turkey bacon (for those more liberal vegetarians who eat fish, chicken, or turkey but not red meat), or soy bacon strips or soy sausage patties. There will be some carbs in the soy alternatives, so you shouldn't indulge in them often during these two weeks. Additionally, you may need to reduce the portions of vegetables or fruits offered to make up the difference during this phase. You'll have much more leeway on the carb front when you move into Weeks 5 and 6 of The Cure.

Besides their added carbohydrate load, however, there's another reason we don't recommend the use of soy products. A widening body of research suggests that processed or precipitated soy, such as soy protein isolate powders, soy milk, bean curd, tofu, and TVP (texturized vegetable protein used to make soy burgers and fake meats), despite their "healthful" reputation might actually be harmful. Anti-nutrients present in processed soy (but destroyed by the long fermentation needed to make tempeh, natto, miso, and tamari) interfere with protein digestion and inhibit the absorption of calcium, magnesium, iron, and zinc. Additionally the plant estrogens in soy products stall or delay sexual development in young boys and accelerate it in young girls. We don't normally recommend processed soy for these reasons. In the case of dieters committed to the vegetarian philosophy, their limited use is probably not problematic in the short term, but it is our opinion that these proteins, damaged as they are by processing and rife with anti-nutrients, offer suboptimal nutrition. It's a trade-off each person must decide to make: optimal nutrition for ideology.

As to lunch and dinner options, if you allow yourself to eat fish, you can substitute any of the fish or seafood dishes (or your favorite ones, as long as they aren't breaded and don't otherwise contain dense sources of carbohydrates) for the beef, pork, lamb, poultry, and game at lunch or dinner. If you eat chicken as well as fish, you'll have lots of options to substitute for meats you don't care to eat. Remember; this phase of the program lasts only two weeks. Where it makes sense to do so, we've also suggested some (albeit less than optimal) vegetarian substitutions to help you along on The Cure.

TAKING STOCK, AGAIN

You've now completed four weeks of The Cure and it's time to take stock of your progress. Repeat your measurements and weight, and jot them down on your Initial Assessment and Progress Log (page 285). If you had initially gotten blood work done by your physician and were concerned before you began The Cure about elevations of blood cholesterol, triglycerides, blood sugar, liver enzymes, or other abnormal blood values, you might now wish to repeat the blood work. You should find those values substantially improved.

Those of you who began The Cure with the typical 10 to 20 excess pounds to be shed from your middle-aged middles should be at or near your goal after four weeks of the regimen. If you determine that your waistline and belly are now as you'd like them to be—in inches, in how you look in the mirror, or in how your clothing fits—it's time to move on to Weeks 5 and 6, and learn how to maintain your leaner middle for life.

Some of you may not quite be there yet. You may have begun with bigger middles than can reasonably be shed in four weeks, or perhaps you're almost there but not quite where you'd like to be. Others of you, however, may have seen your weights remain stable for the last week or so and at this point are wondering, "What in blazes is going on?"

A part of what happens to many people in these first four weeks involves changes in body composition. There's an old joke that goes: What would Mozart be doing if he were here with us today? The groaner of an answer is, "decomposing." What you've been doing for the past four weeks, courtesy of your increased protein intake—and especially increased leucine intake—is *recomposing*.

You've been swapping fat pounds for muscle and bone pounds, but to the scale they all weigh the same. The scale can't differentiate among fat, water, or lean muscle and bone. Weight is weight. So if your weight hasn't dropped during these two weeks as rapidly as it did in the first two weeks, even if it has stabilized, don't despair. Look deeper. How do your clothes fit? How many notches down is your belt? What is your SAD measurement? How much more difference is there between that measurement taken standing and lying down? If you've been faithfully following the guidelines, rest assured that, frustrating as it may be to not see the scale number dropping more quickly, this recomposition is beneficial. Swapping fat for muscle, pound for pound, will hold you in good stead when it comes time to maintain your lean middle for the long haul. Keep the faith and your scale weight will ultimately catch up.

Whatever the reason—recomposition or a longer way to go than can be accomplished in four short weeks—if you're not quite where you want to be, here's what to do: keep going, alternating the first two eating patterns. For a week, follow the eating guidelines of Weeks 1 and 2; for the next week, follow the guidelines of Weeks 3 and 4. This method will prevent you from becoming bored, but will also vary your calorie intake up and down in short windows that prevent the metabolism from going into a starvation panic and ratcheting back its energy expenditure. Alternate between the two regimens, reassessing after each week, until your middle-aged middle is trimmed to your satisfaction. Then move on to Weeks 5 and 6. There's no need to do the complete detox routine again with the total prohibitions on alcohol, caffeine, and medications, but as in the two weeks you've just completed, use common sense and enjoy these reasonably.

8

THE CURE: WEEKS 5 AND 6

"To get back my youth, I would do anything in the world,
except take exercise, get up early, or be respectable."
—Oscar Wilde

The hardest work is over and now it's time to learn how to eat to maintain the slender silhouette you've created, through middle age and beyond. We don't mean to imply that maintaining won't also require some work, dedication, and stick-to-itive-ness to be successful for the long haul, because it surely will. As you approach these last two weeks of The Cure and begin what we'd like you to view as a lifelong healthy eating pattern, we ask you to recognize that maintenance is a journey, not a destination. The stresses and, perhaps even more commonly, the traditions and pleasures of life have a way of occasionally undermining even the most fervently sworn oaths against dietary overindulgence. It's perfectly normal and, we think, emotionally healthy to indulge yourself now and again, but just that— now and again—and with a plan in place to guide you back to metabolic balance. It's certainly how we, ourselves, have lived for the last quarter of a century or so.

There will be times of smooth sailing and of rough waters as you strive to maintain your dietary commitments, just as there are in all facets of life. Your job is to learn to go with the flow, certain in the knowledge that you know what to do, firm in the belief that as long as you continue to feed your body appropriately, you will reap the lasting reward of sounder sleep, increased energy, better health, and a trimmer middle. Let's take a look at how rich and satisfying good nutrition can be.

THE RULES OF THE GAME—WEEKS 5 AND 6

1. *Enjoy moderate alcohol intake, if you so desire.* Moderation, by our definition here, means no more than two drinks (4-ounce glasses of wine, 12-ounce light beers, or single shots of distilled spirits) per day and not necessarily every day.*

2. *You may reintroduce dairy products, such as cheeses, yogurt, sour cream, and sweet cream.* We opt for full-fat products over low-fat ones, although we recommend choosing organic dairy products as much as possible to reduce the toxic load of pesticides, hormones, and growth factors that may concentrate in the fat of the animal's milk (as discussed in Chapter 4).

3. *You may reintroduce starchy vegetables, grains, and things made from them in very limited quantities, if you tolerate them and desire to do so.* During this two-week period of easing into maintenance, limit your intake to no more than 10 to 12 effective (net) grams of grain starch per day. Thereafter you may gingerly ease your carbohydrate intake upward, if you so desire. If you see your weight begin to creep up, cut back. (See box on pages 150–151, "About Concentrated Starches.")

---

* For the long haul, we recommend not drinking every day and taking periodic abstinence periods of 4 or 5 days at least once every three months to give your liver a break.

ABOUT CONCENTRATED STARCHES
(GRAINS, TUBERS, AND LEGUMES)

Remember that grains—even whole grains—are primarily just a source of starch calories and some fiber. And starches are basically just sugars—glucose molecules—hooked in long chains that the digestive tract quickly and easily breaks down. Unless they're fortified, grains aren't especially dense in nutrients and are filled with anti-nutrients and lectins that can promote inflammation. If eaten in excess, these foods can undermine your long-term success in keeping control of your middle. If you can manage without them forever, so much the better for your health and waistline.

Starchy tubers (potatoes, yams) and legumes (dried beans and peas) are a bit more micronutrient-dense, but they are still loaded with carbs easily turned to sugar that can undermine your metabolic balance if eaten too liberally. With all delicious sugary and starchy edibles, portion control and moderation should be your watchwords. As a general rule, during this two-week march to maintenance, you should strive to consume your carbohydrate grams as low-sugar fruits and low-starch vegetables and eat no more than a total of 10 to 12 effective (net) grams of carbohydrate as grain or starchy tubers per day.

Staying within or near that ballpark—10 grams—would mean eating only *one* portion of any *one* of the following foods *once* a day:

- 1 small low-carb tortilla (about 7 grams)
- 1 slice of "light" bread (about 6 or 7 grams)
- 1 "light" hot dog or hamburger bun (about 13 grams)
- ¼ scant cup cooked rice (about 10 grams)
- 6 tablespoons of sushi rice (about 2.5 grams per tablespoon)
- 2 (single) pieces nigiri sushi* (about 5 grams each)
- ⅓ cup cooked oatmeal (about 10 grams)
- 2 cups of plain popped corn (about 5 grams each cup)

* Each single piece of nigiri sushi contains about two tablespoons of rice.

continued

- ¼ cup cooked dried beans (about 10 grams)
- ⅓ medium sweet potato (about 10 grams)
- ¼ cup hashbrown potatoes (about 10 grams)
- ⅓ cup cooked potato (about 9 grams)
- ¼ medium baked potato, including the skin (about 11 grams)

4. Continue to take a daily multiple vitamin and mineral supplement (as in Weeks 3 and 4) as cheap nutritional insurance. As was the case in the previous two weeks, you may continue to take the full Weeks 1 and 2 supplement regimen, if you so desire; it's what we take ourselves, but it's not mandatory for successful maintenance.

Obviously you needn't eat your entire 10 gram maximum allotment of concentrated starch—that is, that from grains, tubers, or legumes—in a single food or in a single meal. You don't have to eat any non-vegetable starch at all, if you'd rather not. If you choose to partake, however, you can mix and match from these foods to enjoy *up to but no more than* a total of 10 to 12 grams of starch from grain, tuber, or legumes in a 24-hour period. Recognize, too, that there are some of you for whom even this much starch will prove a challenge, metabolically and to your appetite. Some people will not be able to eat this much concentrated carbohydrate without shutting down their fat burning. A carbohydrate-gram counting book, such as our *Protein Power LifePlan Gram Counter* (Warner, 2000), will aid you here.

CAVE CARBUM! (BEWARE THE CARBS!)

You will notice as you read through the meal plans for these weeks that we've liberalized the amount of fruits and vegetables that you can enjoy and have even added a few starchier foods. We've specified portion sizes for all the foods for the next two weeks that contain more than a few grams of carbohydrate per serving. Remember that it's the carbohydrate portion of any food that can wreak metabolic havoc and refatten your liver and your waistline. You will maintain your hard-won, flatter, thinner middle only by continuing to keep some measure of control of carbs for the long haul. So how much does that mean?

Actually, the absolute number of total effective (net) carbohydrate grams that someone can eat and still maintain varies, by both the person and the situation. Generally speaking, the more active you are the more carb grams you will likely tolerate and still maintain your weight, health, and waistline. The flip side of that maxim, however, is that if your level of activity drops, so must your carbohydrate intake if you are to maintain your health and leanness.

Our decades of experience tell us that the average person (not totally sedentary, not heavily athletic) will usually tolerate something in the range of 60 to 80 total effective (net) grams per day, but that's nothing more than a ballpark guess. What your metabolism and lifestyle will tolerate is a number you will find out over time. After this first two weeks of prescribed eating, feel free to ease your intake of carbohydrate-containing foods upward as you feel comfortable to the amount at which you just begin to gain a little weight. At that point, you will have exceeded your metabolic tolerance for carbohydrate intake, and you should back down 10 grams per day or so to maintain. Conversely, you could choose to work the other direction of the energy balance equation—that is, becoming more physically active—and maintain that way.

As a rule of thumb, in maintenance, if you stick primarily to the lower sugar fruits (berries, melon, peaches, grapes, apples, oranges, kiwi) and the lower starch vegetables (asparagus, beets, broccoli, cabbage, carrots, cauliflower, celery, celeriac, green beans, greens, lettuces, mushrooms, onion, peppers, squashes, and tomatoes) you will be hard pressed to consume more than 20 grams of effective (net) carbohydrate in a single meal. In maintenance you can enjoy virtually an unlimited amount of these kinds of foods and maintain nicely. It's when you stray into that dense starchy, sugary territory—bananas, breads, tropical fruits, potatoes, dried beans and peas, cereal grains, cakes, pies, cookies, candy, sodas, and other sources of concentrated simple sugars—that portion control becomes key. For instance, a single bagel (which contains about 37 grams of carbohydrate) can gobble up half your day's carb total; it would take 92 spears of asparagus, or 11 cups of broccoli, or 9 tomatoes to equal that carb load. While you'll probably never eat 92 spears of asparagus at a sitting, if you're like us and most of our patients, you could easily imagine scarfing down a bagel without a blink.

We think it's an added bonus that the foods that keep you lean happen also to be the foods that keep you healthy.

THE MAINTENANCE MEAL PLANS

As before, these meal plans are simply suggestions for what you might eat. You can select from the breakfasts, lunches, or dinners freely, mixing and matching them as you craft your day's menu. You may repeat favorites and eschew the ones that don't appeal to you. As before, within any given meal, the mix of carbohydrate-containing foods has been crafted to provide a maximum limit—in this case, under 20 effective (net) grams of carbohydrate. When you design your own maintenance meals, keep this carbohydrate total in mind and add to it an amount of protein and fat-containing foods (meat, fish, poultry, game, eggs, dairy, nuts, seeds, and quality oils) that satisfies your hunger.

If there is a food you cannot eat or do not like, you may again turn to the Fruit and Vegetable Substitution lists in the Appendix to select an alternative.

Suggested Breakfast for Weeks 5 and 6
1. Confetti Omelet,* with crisp bacon (or turkey bacon)
    3 or 4 thick tomato slices, sprinkled with sea salt
    1 slice "light" toast with butter and 1 teaspoon low-sugar jam, if
      desired
    Water, tea, or coffee (caf or decaf)

---

* Recipes can be found in the Recipe section of this book.

2. Oatmeal (½ cup, cooked) with butter, cream, and Splenda or
   stevia, if desired

   ⅛ cup walnut or pecan pieces

   Crisp bacon or sausage patties (turkey or pork)

   Water, tea, or coffee (caf or decaf)

3. Egg and Sausage Pie*

   1 cup Mixed Fruit Salad*

   Water, tea, or coffee (caf or decaf)

4. Goldilox Scramble*

   ½ cup cherry tomato halves, with a sprinkling of capers and
   diced red onion, drizzled with olive oil vinaigrette, if desired

   ½ cup melon cubes with a squeeze of fresh lime juice and a
   sprinkling of lime zest

   Water, tea, or coffee (caf or decaf)

5. Ham and Asparagus Scramble*

   1 small (Valencia) orange, sliced

   Water, tea, or coffee (caf or decaf)

6. Lemon Ricotta Flapjacks* with Sugar-Free Maple Syrup*

   Crisp bacon (turkey or pork)

   1 cup fresh blackberries

   Water, tea, or coffee (caf or decaf)

7. Powered-up Waffle* with melted butter and Sugar-Free Maple
   Syrup*

   2 or 3 links (turkey or pork) sausage

   1 serving Strawberry, Mandarin, and Mint Cup*

   Water, tea, or coffee (caf or decaf)

8. Smoked salmon slices

   2 tablespoons cream cheese

   1 low-carb (or ½ regular) bagel

   1 leaf butter (or other soft head) lettuce

   3 or 4 thin tomato slices and a sprinkling of diced red onion
   and capers

   Water, tea, or coffee (caf or decaf)

9. Poached Eggs on Herbed Broiled Tomato Slices*
   Sausage patties or crisp bacon
   1 slice "light" toast with butter
   ½ cup sautéed spinach
   ½ cup fresh melon
   Water, tea, or coffee (caf or decaf)

10. Powered-up Kefir and Fresh Berries*
    Crisp bacon or sausage patties (turkey or pork)
    Water, tea, or coffee (caf or decaf)

11. Sausage, Egg, and Cheese Scramble*
    ½ cup fresh spinach, sautéed with butter and garlic
    ½ cup fresh berries
    1 warm low-carb tortilla, with butter and 1 teaspoon low-sugar
      jam
    Water, tea, or coffee (caf or decaf)

12. Ham and Asparagus Scramble*
    ½ medium tomato, sliced, salted, and drizzled with
      olive oil
    ⅓ cup hashbrown potatoes
    Water, tea, or coffee (caf or decaf)

13. Poached Eggs on Herbed Broiled Tomato Slices*
    ¼ cup Low-Carb Mornay Sauce*
    Crisp bacon (or turkey bacon) slices
    1 slice "light" toast, with butter
    Water, tea, or coffee (caf or decaf)

14. Deviled Eggs with Lox and Capers*
    ½ avocado, salted, drizzled with balsamic vinaigrette
    1 small (Valencia) orange, sliced
    Water, tea, or coffee (caf or decaf)

15. Scrambled Egg Roll-Ups*
    ½ cup fresh grapes
    1 low-carb tortilla, warm (if desired)
    Water, tea, or coffee (caf or decaf)

16. Florentine Scramble* wrap
    ½ cup fresh grapes
    Water, tea, or coffee (caf or decaf)

17. Eggs, fried in butter
    Crisp bacon
    2 slices tomato, salted
    ½ Hass avocado, sliced, drizzled with olive oil, sprinkled with
        salt and pepper
    1 slice "light" toast, buttered, with 1 teaspoon low-sugar
        jam
    Water, tea, or coffee (caf or decaf)

Suggested Lunches

1. Hamburger pattie(s), on a "light" hamburger bun
    1 or 2 strips crisp bacon or turkey bacon
    ½ Hass avocado, sliced
    1 slice ripe tomato
    1 large lettuce leaf
    Mayo, mustard, dill pickle, as desired
    (Opt for a lettuce-wrapped burger and add a small apple)
    Water, tea, or coffee (caf or decaf)

2. Chili dog with "light" hot dog bun
    Dill pickle relish, mustard, onions, as desired
    ½ cup Crunchy Cabbage Slaw*
    1 or 2 dill pickle spears, if desired
    (Opt for a naked dog and add a Valencia orange)
    Water, tea, or coffee (caf or decaf)

3. Rotisserie chicken (take-out or home-roasted)
    ½ cup Sunny Day Garden Salad*
    ⅓ cup pinto or lima beans
    Water, tea, or coffee (caf or decaf)

4. Gyro Burger(s)* in a small, warm, low-carb tortilla
    ½ cup Mediterranean Chopped Salad*
    ½ small apple, sliced

(Opt for a lettuce-wrapped gyro burger and enjoy a whole apple)

Water, tea, or coffee (caf or decaf)

5. Chicken Caesar Salad Lettuce Wrap(s)*

   1 small (Valencia) orange, sliced

   ½ cup fresh grapes

   Water, tea, or coffee (caf or decaf)

6. Antipasto Lunch Plate*

   2 slices (1-inch) crusty Italian bread with olive oil and balsamic
   vinegar for dipping

   Water, tea, or coffee (caf or decaf)

7. Inside Out Triple-Decker Ham Sandwich(es)*

   ½ cup Crunchy Cabbage Slaw*

   1 small apple, sliced

   Water, tea, or coffee (caf or decaf)

8. Gourmet Nutty Bird Burger(s)* on a "light" hamburger bun

   Mayo, mustard, pickle as desired

   ¼ cup Cranberry-Orange Relish*

   (Opt for a lettuce-wrapped burger and add 1 cup fresh berries
   and ½ cup grapes)

   Water, tea, or coffee (caf or decaf)

9. Thai Chicken Lettuce Wraps*

   1 cup miso soup

   1 small pear, sliced

   Water, tea, or coffee (caf or decaf)

10. Chicken Caesar Salad*

    ½ cup grapes

    1 slice (1-inch) crusty French baguette, with butter, if desired

    Water, tea, or coffee (caf or decaf)

11. Broiled lamb (or beef) burger, on a "light" hamburger bun, if
    desired

    1 cup Mediterranean Chopped Salad*

    2 slices Grilled Halloumi*

    (Opt for a lettuce-wrapped burger and add 1 peach or nectarine)

    Water, tea, or coffee (caf or decaf)

12. 1½ cups Very Chickeny (or Beefy) Vegetable Soup*
    1 slice (1-inch) crusty French baguette, with butter
    1 or 2 ounces hard cheese
    Water, tea, or coffee (caf or decaf)

13. BLAT Lettuce Wrap*
    2 to 3 ounces brie cheese and ½ cup grapes
    Water, tea, or coffee (caf or decaf)

14. Chef's salad (lettuce, broccoli florets, red onion, grated carrot,
    diced tomato, hard-boiled egg with choice of diced ham,
    turkey, or chicken and crumbled bacon, if desired, and grated
    Cheddar or crumbled feta or blue cheese)
    1 slice (1-inch) crusty French baguette, with butter
    Ranch, blue cheese, or olive oil vinaigrette dressing
    Water, tea, or coffee (caf or decaf)

15. Buffalo Chicken Wings*
    Salad of mixed greens with bleu cheese dressing (or choice)
    ½ cup each carrot and celery sticks and broccoli or cauliflower
    florets
    ½ cup mixed berries with a dollop of artificially sweetened
    whipped cream
    Water, tea, or coffee (caf or decaf)

16. Chicken (or Tuna) Salad Stuffed Tomato* with olive oil
    vinaigrette
    ½ small apple
    4 or 5 Blue Diamond Almond Nut Thin crackers
    1 or 2 ounces Cheddar or Monterey jack cheese
    Water, tea, or coffee (caf or decaf)

17. Classic Cobb Salad* with blue cheese or other dressing of your
    choice
    5 or 6 Blue Diamond Almond Nut Thin Crackers (or 3 or 4
    saltines) with butter
    ½ cup grapes for dessert
    Water, tea, or coffee (caf or decaf)

18. Grilled chicken breast on a "light" hamburger bun
Mayo, mustard, ketchup, and pickle, as desired
2 cups mixed green salad, with olive oil vinaigrette
(Opt for a lettuce-wrapped sandwich and add 1 small orange or
    tangerine)
Water, tea, or coffee (caf or decaf)

Suggested Dinners Weeks 5 and 6

1. Grilled Citrus-Rosemary Salmon*
    4 or 5 roasted asparagus spears, with butter, salt, and
        pepper
    ½ cup Cauliflower Puree*
    ½ cup fresh berries, with a dollop of whipped cream
    Water, tea, or coffee (caf or decaf)
2. Lamb and Red Pepper Kebabs*
    1 cup salad greens with olive oil vinaigrette
    1 serving Parmesan Broccoli and Red Peppers*
    1 serving Savory Sautéed Apple Slices* with a dollop of
        unsweetened whipped cream
    Water, tea, or coffee (caf or decaf)
3. Grilled Spice-Rubbed Flank Steak*
    1 cup sautéed broccoli with butter, garlic, salt, and pepper
    1 medium tomato, in wedges, with olive oil vinaigrette
    1 Grilled Plum*
    Water, tea, or coffee (caf or decaf)
4. Chicken with 40 Cloves of Garlic*
    1 cup Herbed Cauli-Rice*
    1 cup Mediterranean Chopped Salad*
    ½ small (Valencia) orange, sliced
    Water, tea, or coffee (caf or decaf)
5. Fish and Peppers Packets*
    ½ cup sautéed zucchini, drizzled with olive oil and balsamic
        vinegar

1 cup mixed lettuces, with olive oil vinaigrette or your choice of
    dressing
1 serving Savory Sautéed Apple Slices*
Water, tea, or coffee (caf or decaf)

6. Speedy Garlic Shrimp*
    1 cup Warm Sesame and Ginger Spinach Salad*
    ½ Hass avocado, sliced, sprinkled with lemon juice, salt, and
        pepper
    2 slices (1-inch) crusty French baguette, with butter
    Water, tea, or coffee (caf or decaf)

7. Triple-Threat Meatloaf*
    ½ cup green beans, seasoned with butter, salt, and pepper
    ½ cup Creamy Cauliflower Puree*
    1 Guilt-free Mini-Cheesecake*
    Water, tea, or coffee (caf or decaf)

8. Grilled steak
    1 serving Parmesan Broccoli and Red Peppers*
    ½ cup Cauliflower Puree*
    ½ cup fresh berries, with a dollop of whipped cream, if desired
    Water, tea, or coffee (caf or decaf)

9. Garlic-Rubbed Pork Tenderloin*
    ½ cup Sautéed Apples and Red Cabbage*
    ½ cup Olive Salad*
    ½ Grilled Plum*
    Water, tea, or coffee (caf or decaf)

10. Lemon Chicken*
    ½ cup Herbed Cauli-Rice*
    ½ cup Greek Salad*
    1 Guilt-free Mini-Cheesecake*
    Water, tea, or coffee (caf or decaf)

11. Herb-Roasted Chicken*
    ⅓ cup buttered baby carrots
    1 cup fresh spinach, sautéed in butter, olive oil, and garlic

½ cup fresh or frozen raspberries topped with Sweet Lime
    Cream*

Water, tea, or coffee (caf or decaf)

12. Grilled Spice-Rubbed Flank Steak*

4 or 5 fresh asparagus spears, steamed, topped with butter, salt,
    and pepper

1 medium tomato, sliced, sprinkled with sea salt (drizzle with
    olive oil and balsamic vinegar, if desired)

½ cup fresh or frozen blackberries, with a dollop of whipped
    cream, if desired

Water, tea, or coffee (caf or decaf)

13. Grilled Citrus-Rosemary Salmon*

½ cup cauliflower florets, steamed, topped with butter, garlic,
    and soy sauce

1 Broiled Herbed Tomato Half*

1 cup fresh mixed lettuces, dressed with balsamic
    vinaigrette

½ Grilled Peach* (Topped with a dollop of artifically sweetened
    whipped cream, if desired)

Water, tea, or coffee (caf or decaf)

14. Garlic-Rubbed Pork Tenderloin*

½ cup Sautéed Apples and Red Cabbage*

4 or 5 spears roasted or steamed asparagus with olive oil, salt,
    and pepper

1 serving Savory Sautéed Apple Slices*

Water, tea, or coffee (caf or decaf)

15. Grilled Herb-Crusted Lamb T-Bones*

4 to 5 spears roasted asparagus

1 cup Mediterranean Chopped Salad*

2 slices of Grilled Halloumi*

½ cup fresh strawberries with (artificially) sweetened whipped
    cream

Water, tea, or coffee (caf or decaf)

16. Triple-Threat Meatloaf*

    ½ cup Creamy Cauliflower Puree*

    ½ cup fresh or frozen green peas, with butter, salt, and pepper

    1 serving Savory Sautéed Apple Slices*

    Water, tea, or coffee (caf or decaf)

17. Lamb and Red Pepper Kebab* on a bed of Herbed Cauli-Rice*

    1 cup Greek Salad* with Minted Yogurt Dressing*

    ½ fresh pear, sliced, with 1 ounce blue cheese

    Water, tea, or coffee (caf or decaf)

18. Grilled steak, any cut

    5 or 6 spears roasted asparagus sprinkled with salt and drizzled
       with olive oil

    ½ cup Creamy Cauliflower Puree*

    4 or 5 steamed baby carrots, sprinkled with olive oil, rosemary,
       and sea salt

    1 cup fresh strawberries, with a dollop of whipped cream, if
       desired

    Water, tea, or coffee (caf or decaf)

19. Roast Pork and Veggie Stir-Fry*

    1 package San-J White Miso Soup with Tofu and Scallions

    1 cup Fried Cauli-Rice*

    Water, tea, or coffee (caf or decaf)

20. Stuffed Buffalo (or Beef) Burgers* on a "light" hamburger bun

    ½ cup Sunny Day Garden Salad* with dressing of your choice

    ½ small (Valencia) orange, sliced

    (Opt for a lettuce-wrapped burger and enjoy a whole orange and
       a whole cup of the salad)

    Water, tea, or coffee (caf or decaf)

21. Beer-Can Chicken*

    ½ cup Creamy Cauliflower Puree*

    ½ cup broccolini (baby broccoli) sautéed in butter with garlic,
       salt, and pepper

    3 or 4 tomato slices sprinkled with sea salt and a drizzle of
       olive oil

1 serving Strawberry, Mandarin, and Mint Cup*

Water, tea, or coffee (caf or decaf)

22. Speedy Garlic Shrimp*

½ cup steamed spaghetti squash tossed with olive oil, salt, and pepper

½ cup Parmesan Broccoli and Red Peppers*

1 slice (1-inch) crusty French baguette, with butter

Water, mineral water, aspartame-free diet soda, coffee or tea

WHAT TO EXPECT NOW

As you did following the previous two phases of this regimen, you should take stock of where you are by weighing and measuring yourself, repeating any laboratory tests that track health issues of concern to you and recording your results in your Initial Assessment and Progress Log (page 285). You may be down a few more pounds, trimmer by a few more inches in your waist, and enjoying a flatter, leaner, younger-looking middle. At the end of this final two-week period of The Cure, your weight may have stabilized—that is, you are probably not continuing to lose weight.

If you are continuing to lose weight on the regimen prescribed in Weeks 5 and 6 of The Cure—and you're at the weight and size you'd like to be—you have two options. You can increase your calories by eating more calorie-dense, carbohydrate-lean foods, such as nuts, olives, avocados, organic dairy, and quality oils, such as olive oil, coconut oil, and butter. These foods will allow you to increase your calories to a maintenance level without raising your insulin level, which could send an unwanted fat-storage signal. Or, you can slightly increase your carbohydrate intake by eating more portions of fruits, vegetables, and, if necessary, grains. We recommend the former option as the healthier one from a metabolic standpoint, but either will stabilize your weight. Be especially judicious if you select the adding-carbs option, however, since your history has proved that taking in a big carb load will send your insulin level skyrocketing and throw the fat-storage switch to the on position. Take your time easing into a maintenance level of carb intake that suits you; add an additional 5- or 10-gram portion of carbohydrate to your daily intake and hold steady there for five to seven days to see how your weight responds. If your weight is still dropping, add another portion. Stop when your weight stabilizes.

If you're anything like us, our family, friends, patients, and readers who have used the plan successfully, you will feel like you've shed ten years in six weeks. And in a sense, you have. You've become substantially leaner, metabolically cleaner, much healthier, and back in balance. Your job now is to maintain that balance. You can do that by continuing to eat a diet much like the one you've enjoyed these last two weeks—one filled with high-quality nutrition from meat, fish, poultry, game, eggs, and dairy; fresh low-starch vegetables and low-sugar fruits; and nuts and seeds—but limited in concentrated starches and sugars. You can throw in the *occasional* dietary vacation purely for pleasure: share a warm Danish; enjoy a double cappuccino, a decadent dessert after a fine meal, cookies at the holidays, or fresh strawberry shortcake at a summer barbecue. Take note, however, that the operative word in that sentence is *occasional*. Dietary vacations that occur too frequently turn into a lifestyle of dietary excess not in keeping with maintaining a slender middle. Make your dietary vacation count: plan for it, look forward to it, and enjoy it. Then get right back to your maintenance plan.

Another option is to alternate every other day between your healthy, maintenance-level diet (as described in this chapter for Weeks 5 and 6) and the 3-and-1 shake plan described in Weeks 1 and 2. Many of our patients and readers have found this option to be easy and they remark that it fits in nicely with their lifestyle. It's just so quick and easy (and foolproof) to whip up a shake. A third option is to replace a single meal each day in maintenance with a Power Up! Protein Shake. Recent medical research has shown that people following this kind of maintenance method re-gain far less weight than those who eat three meals a day, where choices can sometimes undermine good intentions, and further that they may actually lose a few pounds in the course of the year. Select whichever method suits you and your lifestyle best; make a plan that you can stick with over the long haul and you will be rewarded with a lean middle far beyond middle age.

WHAT IF YOU SLIP OFF THE WAGON?

If, in the future, you should find yourself sliding down the dietary slippery slope and your middle begins to expand, don't panic. Take stock of where you are and recall all you've learned about why this weight gain occurs and the various steps you now know can reverse it. The dietary tools you've learned in the preceding weeks will be interventions you can fall back on if you need them in the months and years ahead to reset your metabolic balance once again.

Since we whittled down our own middles using this method several years ago, we have used each of these tools—the 3-and-1 shake week without alcohol and the meat diet week with or without alcohol—to get ourselves back into balance after a vacation or the holidays. A week or so of abstinence from alcohol now and then does a world of good for your liver and, as you now know, a healthy, fat-free liver is your ticket to a lean middle.

In the first year or so following your rehabilitation with The Cure, we recommend that you take stock simply for the sake of doing so, even if things seem stable. Measure and weigh yourself again and enter your results into your Initial Assessment and Progress Log (page 285). Then, even if you are in good shape, about once a quarter—winter, spring, summer, and fall work well—select one of the two dietary tools of The Cure to follow for a week. Call it "The Prophylaxis." This re-centering method will keep you from rolling too far down the hill if you happen to fall off the maintenance wagon. If you find yourself so far out of balance that a week of strict compliance with one of these dietary prescriptions won't be enough to get the job done, take an honest look at where you are and begin The Cure again, working it just as you did before.

Detox your liver and do the full two weeks of each phase, and you'll be right back on track in no time.

We designed this program to be a diet you can live with, one that provides you with a healthy and nutritious eating plan you can use every day from here on out and a pair of tools you can use for years to come to keep your middle well trimmed. With The Cure, "middle-aged" will no longer be a description of your shape; it will just be a number.

RECIPES

EGGS AND OTHER BREAKFAST DISHES

Power Up! Protein Shake

Asparagus and Bacon Crustless Quiche

Confetti Omelet

Deviled Eggs with Lox and Capers

Egg and Sausage Pie

Sausage, Egg, and Cheese Scramble

Florentine Scramble

Goldilox Scramble

Ham and Asparagus Scramble

Scrambled Egg Roll-Up

Poached Eggs on Herbed Broiled Tomato Slices

Grilled (or Griddled) Halloumi

Lemon Ricotta Flapjacks

Sugar-Free Maple Syrup

Powered-up Waffles

Powered-up Kefir and Fresh Berries

Strawberry Blues Protein Smoothie

SOUPS AND SALADS

Very Chickeny (or Beefy) Vegetable Soup

Meat Week Soup

BLAT Lettuce Wraps

Chicken Caesar Salad Lettuce Wraps

Chicken Club Salad Lettuce Wraps

Simple Caesar Salad

Classic Cobb Salad

Greek Salad

Grilled Chicken Salad

Chicken (or Tuna) Salad Stuffed Tomato

Mediterranean Chopped Salad
Olive Salad
Sunny Day Garden Salad
Warm Sesame and Ginger Spinach Salad

BEEF, PORK, AND LAMB

Antipasto Lunch Plate
Beef Tenderloin and Asparagus Roll-Ups
Garlic-Rubbed Beef Tenderloin
Roast Pork and Veggie Stir-Fry
Grilled Herb-Crusted Lamb T-Bones
Rosemary and Mint Rack of Lamb
Grilled Spice-Rubbed Flank Steak
Gyro Burgers
Inside Out Triple-Decker Ham Sandwich
Lamb and Red Pepper Kebabs
Meat Week Chili
Pork Tenderloin Roast
Stuffed Buffalo (or Beef) Burgers
Triple-Threat Meatloaf

CHICKEN AND POULTRY

Beer-Can Chicken
Buffalo Chicken Wings
Chicken Mushroom Packets
Chicken with 40 Cloves of Garlic
Gourmet Nutty Bird Burgers
Herb-Roasted Chicken
Lemon Chicken

Macadamia-Crusted Chicken Paillard
Thai Chicken Lettuce Wraps

FISH AND SEAFOOD

Ahi Tuna Tartare
Baked Salsa Snapper
Cioppino (Fisherman's Stew)
Fish and Peppers Packets
Seared Ahi Tuna
Grilled Citrus-Rosemary Salmon
Shrimp Salad–Stuffed Avocado
Speedy Garlic Shrimp

VEGETABLES AND FRUITS

Broccoli Amondine
Parmesan Broccoli and Red Peppers
Broiled Herbed Tomato Halves
Honey-Mustard Green Beans
Creamy Cauliflower Puree
Fried Cauli-Rice
Herbed Cauli-Rice
Crunchy Cabbage Slaw
Sautéed Apples and Red Cabbage
Savory Sautéed Apple Slices
Grilled Plums, Nectarines, or Peaches
Chilled Fruit Soup
Sweet Orange Water
Strawberry, Mandarin, and Mint Cup
Mixed Fruit Salad

JUST A FEW SWEET TREATS

Homemade Vanilla Ice Cream
Guilt-free Mini-Cheesecakes
Sweet Lime Cream

SAUCES, CONDIMENTS, AND DRESSINGS

Basic Blender Mayonnaise
Caesar Dressing
Creamy Gorgonzola Dressing
Minted Yogurt Dressing
Dijon Vinaigrette
Minted Vinegar
Low-Carb Béchamel Sauce
Cranberry-Orange Relish

EGGS AND OTHER
BREAKFAST DISHES

POWER UP! PROTEIN SHAKE

Serves 1

See Resources for recommended products and online sources for protein powders, leucine, and D-ribose.

¾ cups (6 ounces) cold water
1 packet Splenda, stevia, xylitol, or erythritol sweetener (optional)
2 tablespoons heavy cream (organic if possible) or premium coconut milk
Flavorings as desired (see pages 119–120)
1 to 3* scoops low-carb whey protein powder (any flavor)
2500 mg leucine (in branch-chain amino acid supplement capsules or powder)
2500 mg D-ribose powder (optional)
Approximately 1 cup ice cubes

1. Place all the ingredients in a blender in the order above and blend on high speed until smooth.

2. Adjust the amount of ice to achieve preferred consistency. Drink immediately.

Note: You can also make a thinner version of the shake by shaking ingredients in a tightly sealed, lidded container if no blender is available. The ice will chill the shake, but won't be crushed to make it thick.

---

* The amount of protein in these products varies. Most contain 18–22 grams per scoop. People under 130 pounds should use 1 scoop, those 131–180 should use 2 scoops, and those 181 and over should use 3 scoops.

ASPARAGUS AND BACON
CRUSTLESS QUICHE

Serves 4

8 asparagus spears

2 tablespoons butter

¼ quarter small onion, diced

6 large eggs

4 slices bacon, cooked until crisp and crumbled

½ cup shredded Cheddar, Monterey jack, or similar cheese

⅛ teaspoon garlic powder

⅛ teaspoon paprika

Salt and pepper to taste

1. Preheat the oven to 350° F.

2. Snap the white ends off the asparagus and trim green tips to 4-inch lengths. Place in a microwave-safe dish, cover with 1 tablespoon water, and microwave on high for 2 minutes (or place in boiling water and boil for 2 minutes).

3. Melt the butter in a medium ovenproof sauté pan or skillet over medium heat. Add the onion and sauté until translucent, about 3 minutes.

4. Beat the eggs well, and add the bacon, cheese, and seasonings. Pour the egg mixture into the sauté pan. Arrange the asparagus spears like spokes in a wheel with the tips pointing outward.

5. Place the skillet in the oven and bake for 30 minutes, until puffed up and golden brown. Slice and serve.

Meat Week Variation: Omit the cheese and add ½ cup thawed frozen spinach, squeezed dry of liquid.

Time-saving Tip: Make two pies at once. Cool and wrap the individual wedges in plastic. Remove plastic wrap, place in a microwave-safe dish, and cover with a paper towel. Reheat in the microwave for about 2 minutes on 80 percent power and then in 30-second bursts on high until heated through.

Vegetarian Option: Substitute turkey or soy bacon for the pork bacon.

CONFETTI OMELET

Serves 1

3 large eggs
2 tablespoons butter
1 tablespoon finely diced red bell pepper
1 tablespoon finely diced green bell pepper
1 tablespoon finely diced yellow bell pepper
1 tablespoon finely diced white onion
Salt and pepper to taste

1. In a bowl, beat the eggs until pale and frothy.

2. Melt the butter in a nonstick skillet or omelet pan over medium-high heat. Do not let the butter burn. Sauté the diced peppers and onion until softened, about 3 minutes.

3. Add the eggs and allow them to cook, undisturbed, for a couple of minutes, then flip the omelet and cook on the other side. (Or, instead of flipping, use a flexible spatula to gently lift the edges of the omelet to allow the liquid egg to run underneath. Work your way around the pan until no liquid egg remains.)

4. Fold the omelet in half and slide onto the serving plate. Serve.

Maintenance Variation: Add 2 tablespoons shredded cheese to the beaten eggs, if desired.

DEVILED EGGS WITH LOX AND CAPERS

Serves 4

4 large eggs

2 ounces smoked salmon lox or Nova Scotia salmon

2 tablespoons Basic Blender Mayonnaise (page 272)

2 teaspoons Dijon mustard

1 tablespoon dill pickle juice

¼ teaspoon salt

¼ teaspoon black pepper

⅛ teaspoon garlic powder

Sprinkle of paprika

1 tablespoon drained capers

1. Place the eggs in a small saucepan and add enough cold water to cover them. Bring to a boil, remove from the heat, cover, and leave them in the hot water for 10 minutes. Cool under running water, then peel the eggs.

2. Cut the hard-boiled eggs in half and remove the yolks to a bowl; set the white halves aside.

3. Dice the salmon finely and set aside.

4. Mash the yolks with a fork and add the mayonnaise, mustard, pickle juice, and seasonings, except paprika. Fold in the capers and salmon.

5. Fill each egg half with a scoop of the yolk mixture. Add a sprinkling of paprika to each egg for color.

EGG AND SAUSAGE PIE

Serves 4

1 tablespoon butter, plus a bit more for greasing pan

8 ounces Italian mild or hot sausage, removed from casings and
     crumbled

3 large eggs

2 tablespoons chopped fresh parsley, or 2 teaspoons dried

Salt and pepper to taste

¾ cup grated Cheddar or Monterey jack cheese, or combination

1. Preheat the oven to 350° F. Lightly butter a 9-inch pie pan or casserole dish.

2. In a skillet, melt the tablespoon of butter over medium heat. Add the sausage, breaking it up with the spatula or spoon as you cook into very small, even pieces. Brown the meat, drain, and let rest until cool enough to handle.

3. Press the sausage meat into the pie plate and spread out as you would for a piecrust to the edges and slightly up the sides.

4. Break the eggs over the sausage, keeping yolks intact. Sprinkle about half the parsley over the eggs; add a touch of salt and pepper (not too much; the sausage will add some of both).

5. Bake the eggs until the whites are almost set, 7 to 8 minutes.

6. Remove pie from the oven, sprinkle on the cheese, and return to the oven until cheese is melted, 6 or 7 minutes more. Top pie with the remaining parsley, cut into wedges, and serve.

Meat Week Variation: Omit the cheese topping.

Vegetarian Option: Replace the sausage with 8 ounces ground turkey (for those who will eat poultry) or 4 thawed veggie burger patties, crumbled. Season the turkey or veggie burger with ¼ teaspoon dried sage, ⅛ teaspoon black pepper, ⅛ teaspoon garlic powder, ⅛ teaspoon onion powder, ⅛ teaspoon dried ginger, and ⅛ teaspoon crushed red pepper flakes to give it more of a sausage flavor.

Time-saving tip: Make the pie without the cheese topping and slice it into wedges. When cool, wrap the pie plate tightly with plastic and refrigerate for up to 3 days. To reheat, top a slice with cheese, cover with waxed paper, and microwave for 2 minutes on 80 percent power, then in 30-second bursts on high until the cheese is melted and pie is heated through.

SAUSAGE, EGG, AND CHEESE SCRAMBLE

Serves 1

This recipe can easily be doubled or otherwise increased to serve more. Also, alter the number of eggs depending on your appetite and size; smaller people use 2, larger people use 4, those in the middle use 3.

1 tablespoon butter

1 to 2 ounces breakfast patty sausage

2 to 4 large eggs, well beaten

2 tablespoons grated Mexican cheese

Salt and pepper to taste

1. Melt the butter in a skillet over medium heat.

2. Crumble the sausage into the pan and brown evenly, about 5 minutes.

3. Add the beaten eggs, salt, and pepper.

4. Scramble eggs to desired doneness, stirring often to prevent sticking, 3 to 4 minutes. Add the cheese on top and serve.

Meat Week Variation: Omit the cheese and add an ounce more sausage.

Vegetarian Option: Replace the sausage with ground turkey (if acceptable) or 1 veggie burger patty, crumbled, and spice with a dash each of paprika, garlic powder, onion powder, and dried sage.

FLORENTINE SCRAMBLE

Serves 2

4 or 5 large eggs

½ package (10-ounces) frozen chopped spinach, thawed

¼ teaspoon salt

¼ teaspoon black pepper

Dash of freshly grated nutmeg (2 or 3 swipes across the grater)

1 tablespoon olive oil

2 tablespoons diced onion

1 garlic clove, minced

1. In a bowl, beat the eggs until foamy and set aside.

2. Put the spinach in a clean kitchen towel, bring all the corners together, and twist tightly to wring out all the moisture (it will stain the towel, so use an old one).

3. Add the spinach and the seasonings to the eggs and stir to combine.

4. In a skillet, heat the olive oil over medium heat. Add the onion and sauté until translucent, about 3 minutes. Add the garlic and sauté another minute or so.

5. Add the egg mixture to the skillet, stir to combine with the onion and garlic, and cook over medium heat, stirring often to prevent sticking, until the eggs are cooked to your liking, 3 to 4 minutes. Serve at once.

Flavor Variation: Add 2 slices crisply cooked pancetta, crumbled, and/or ¼ cup grated Parmesan cheese to the egg mixture.

GOLDILOX SCRAMBLE

Serves 2

4 to 6 large eggs

2 to 3 ounces cream cheese, softened

4 ounces smoked salmon, diced

Pinch of salt and pepper

2 tablespoons butter

1 tablespoon diced white onion

1 tablespoon diced ripe tomato

1 tablespoon drained capers

1. Beat the eggs well, add the cream cheese and salmon, and season with a pinch of salt and pepper.

2. Melt the butter over medium heat in a small skillet. Add the onion and sauté until translucent, about 3 minutes. Add the egg mixture and stir to prevent sticking, until the eggs are cooked to desired doneness, about 3 to 4 minutes more.

3. Sprinkle the diced tomatos and capers over the top and serve.

Meat Week Variation: Omit the cream cheese.

HAM AND ASPARAGUS SCRAMBLE

Serves 2

2 tablespoons butter

4 asparagus spears, washed, trimmed, and cut into 1-inch pieces

4 ounces cooked ham, diced (½ cup)

4 large eggs

⅛ teaspoon garlic powder

⅛ teaspoon paprika

Salt and pepper to taste

1. In a skillet, melt the butter over medium heat. Add the asparagus pieces and sauté until tender, 2½ to 3 minutes, then add the ham and continue cooking.

2. In a bowl, beat the eggs well. Add the seasonings and beat again.

3. Pour the beaten eggs into the skillet and fold to combine with the ham and asparagus, stirring to prevent sticking. Cook until the eggs are set or to your desired level of doneness, about 3 to 4 minutes more.

4. Divide evenly between two plates and serve.

Maintenance Variation: Add ¼ cup shredded Swiss or fontina cheese to the egg mixture in the pan.

Vegetarian Option: Omit the ham; if desired, replace with 2 ounces smoked salmon (if you eat fish) or 2 ounces diced baked tofu.

SCRAMBLED EGG ROLL-UP

Serves 1 or 2

4 large eggs

1 teaspoon chopped fresh parsley, or ¼ teaspoon dried

⅛ teaspoon garlic powder

⅛ teaspoon onion powder

Sea salt and ground black pepper to taste

4 breakfast sausage links (hot or mild)

2 tablespoons butter

1. Beat the eggs well and stir in the seasonings. Set aside.

2. In a medium nonstick skillet, brown the sausage links until heated through, about 5 minutes. Remove to paper towels to drain.

3. Melt the butter in the same skillet, swirling to coat the surface. Add the eggs and allow them to cook, undisturbed, for a minute or two. Then as if making an omelet, gently lift the edges and tip the pan to let uncooked egg flow underneath, repeating until no liquid egg remains and the surface is nearly cooked, about 3 minutes.

4. Lay the 4 sausage links in pairs, end to end, across the near edge of the omelet. With your spatula, roll the cooked eggs around the sausage links and continue rolling to the far side. Remove from the pan and let cool slightly.

5. Wrap the rolled omelet in parchment or waxed paper for a neater-to-eat "to go" meal, or cut roll in half and serve.

Maintenance Variation: Add 2 tablespoons shredded cheese or diced cream cheese on top of the meat before rolling. Top with hot or mild salsa, if desired.

Vegetarian Variation: Substitute veggie links for sausage.

Time-saver Tip: Make several roll-ups one after the other. Cool, wrap in parchment, then in foil or plastic wrap. Store in a zip closure bag in the refrigerator for up to 3 days. Reheat in parchment only for 2 minutes on 80 percent power, then 30-second blasts on high power until heated through, if needed.

POACHED EGGS ON
HERBED BROILED TOMATO SLICES

Serves 2

FOR THE EGGS

Pinch of coarse salt

1 large ripe tomato

1 teaspoon olive oil

Pinch of Herbes de Provence

Pinch of black pepper

2 slices Canadian bacon

4 large eggs

FOR THE CHEESE SAUCE

½ cup half-and-half

Pinch of salt

Pinch of paprika

Pinch of black pepper

½ cup shredded pepper jack or white Cheddar cheese

1. Prepare the cheese sauce: Warm the half-and-half, salt, paprika, and pepper in a small saucepan over low heat. Just as the cream begins to send up tendrils of steam, stir in the cheese and allow it to melt completely. Keep warm over low heat until ready to serve.

2. Prepare the eggs: Bring 4 cups of water to a boil in a large saucepan. Add a pinch of salt and keep at a simmer.

3. Meanwhile, cut the tomato into 4 thick slices, drizzle with the olive oil, and sprinkle lightly with salt, pepper, and Herbes de Provence.

4. Place the bacon slices on a microwave-safe plate, cover with a paper towel, and warm on high for 30 to 40 seconds.

5. Place the sliced tomatoes on a baking sheet and broil on high for 3 or 4 minutes, or until softened and beginning to brown very slightly.

6. Crack the eggs and slip them into the simmering water, poach for

3 minutes or until the whites are set and the yolks are to desired doneness.

7. Place 2 slices of tomato on each plate and top each with a slice of bacon, a poached egg, and a generous drizzle of cheese sauce.

Meat Week Variation: Omit the cheese sauce.

Vegetarian Option: Omit the bacon or substitute a couple of slices of turkey bacon (if acceptable) or a soy-based bacon substitute.

GRILLED (OR GRIDDLED) HALLOUMI

Serves 2

Halloumi is a cheese from Cyprus, available at many grocery store cheese counters. The cheese does not melt when grilled or heated on a griddle, making it perfect for this application.

4 to 6 slices Halloumi cheese, about ¼ inch thick (4 ounces)
Sugar-Free Maple Syrup (page 189) or low-carb maple syrup

1. Preheat a griddle or grill to medium-hot.
2. Lay the cheese slices on the dry griddle or grate and grill for about 2 minutes. Turn over and grill the other side, as you would a pancake, until golden brown.
3. Serve topped with maple syrup.

Flavor Variation: Sprinkle the cheese slices on both sides with garlic powder, onion powder, dried thyme, and oregano before grilling, for a savory accompaniment to a salad or as an antipasto.

LEMON RICOTTA FLAPJACKS

Serves 4

3 large eggs
1½ cups ricotta cheese
½ cup sour cream
4 packets Splenda, stevia, or erythritol
Juice and zest of 1 large lemon
¼ teaspoon baking soda
½ cup almond flour
¼ cup natural or vanilla whey protein powder
Pinch of salt
1 tablespoon butter
Sugar-Free Maple Syrup (recipe follows), or fresh berries (optional)

1. Preheat a griddle or large skillet over medium-low heat.

2. In a bowl, beat the eggs until light yellow and thick. Beat in the ricotta, sour cream, sweetener, and lemon juice and zest until well combined.

3. In another bowl, combine the dry ingredients. By hand, stir the dry ingredients into the ricotta mixture just until fully blended. Do not over-mix or the flapjacks will be tough.

4. Melt the butter in the skillet. When it foams, ladle the batter by heaping tablespoonfuls, allowing it to spread slightly. Cook in batches to prevent crowding. Cook the flapjacks for 3 to 4 minutes, until golden brown on the bottom and slightly dry on the top; flip and cook until golden brown on the other side, another 2 to 3 minutes.

5. Serve immediately with a bit more butter and the maple syrup or berries, as desired.

SUGAR-FREE MAPLE SYRUP

Makes 1 cup (for about 4 servings)

ThickenThin not/Sugar thickener is both a texturizer that mocks the mouth-feel of sugar and also a gentle thickener. It's a great way to make low-carb gluten-free syrups, jams, and sweet sauces. It's available in some specialty food stores and online at www.proteinpower.com.

1 cup water

1 cup granular Splenda

2 teaspoons maple flavoring (extract)

½ teaspoon ThickenThin not/Sugar thickener or, less optimally, xanthan gum

Place the water, Splenda, and flavoring in a small saucepan. Add the thickener, whisking constantly to prevent clumping. Bring the mixture to a gentle boil over medium-high heat and boil for 1 minute. Serve warm.

Note: Store leftover syrup in a container with a tight-fitting lid in the refrigerator for up to 2 weeks. Reheat gently in the microwave (if in a microwave-safe container) or in a saucepan on the stove.

POWERED-UP WAFFLES

Serves 6

1 cup almond flour or meal
½ cup natural or vanilla whey protein powder
1 teaspoon baking powder
4 ounces cream cheese, softened
6 large eggs
¼ cup heavy cream
Melted butter, for serving
Sugar-Free Maple Syrup (page 189)

1. Preheat a waffle iron, oiling if necessary to prevent sticking.

2. Mix the almond flour, protein powder, and baking powder in a small bowl.

3. Beat the cream cheese until smooth, then beat in the eggs, one at a time, until fully mixed. Beat in the heavy cream. Fold in the dry ingredients, stirring just until combined. Do not overmix or the waffles will be tough.

4. Spoon about ⅓ cup of the batter into the hot waffle iron and cook for about 3 minutes, until golden brown, or according to the manufacturer's instructions.

5. Remove the waffle to a serving plate, and repeat for remaining waffles. Keep cooked waffles warm in a pie plate in the oven on 200°.

6. To serve, top with a bit of melted butter and the maple syrup.

Note: You can cool any leftovers, wrap them in paper towels, put into a zipper-lock freezer bag, and store in the refrigerator for up to 1 week or in the freezer for up to 1 month. To reheat, place the waffles, still wrapped in paper towels, in the microwave and heat on high in 30-second bursts until hot and tender. They can also be reheated in the toaster (without the paper towels, of course).

POWERED-UP KEFIR AND FRESH BERRIES

Serves 1

This recipe can easily be doubled or tripled for multiple servings.

½ cup whole-milk kefir (4 ounces) ·

1 to 3 scoops vanilla low-carb whey protein powder*

½ cup fresh raspberries, cleaned, or strawberries, cleaned, stemmed,
*   and sliced*

1 tablespoon chopped pecans or walnuts

1. In a small bowl, mix the kefir and the protein powder, stirring until smooth. Add a bit of water to thin the mixture if it becomes too thick to pour.

2. Place the berries in a bowl, pour the kefir mixture over them, and top with the chopped nuts.

---

* Most protein powders contain about 18 to 20 grams of protein per scoop. People weighing under 130 pounds, use 1 scoop, those between 130 and 180 use 2 scoops, and those about 180 use 3 scoops. For the list of recommended powders, please see the Appendix.

STRAWBERRY BLUES PROTEIN SMOOTHIE

Serves 1

This is another recipe that is easily multiplied to yield more servings.

½ cup frozen unsweetened blueberries

½ cup ice cubes

1 to 3 scoops strawberry-flavored low-carb whey protein powder

1 cup water

2 tablespoons heavy cream or premium coconut milk

1 packet Splenda, stevia, or erythritol (optional)

1. Place all the ingredients in a blender and put cap on tightly. Pulse to mix, then blend on high speed until smooth.

2. Pour into a tall glass and serve immediately.

Flavor variation: Use ½ blackberries and ½ blueberries and vanilla protein powder for a Black 'n' Blue Smoothie.

VERY CHICKENY (OR BEEFY) VEGETABLE SOUP

Serves 4

1 pound chicken tenders (or lean beef stew meat)
Salt and freshly ground pepper
½ small yellow onion, finely diced
2 tablespoons olive oil
1 garlic clove, finely diced
1 small carrot, finely diced
2 celery stalks, finely diced
1 medium (or 2 small) zucchini, diced
1 can (14 ounces) diced tomatoes with seasoning (basil/onion,
    onion/garlic, Italian seasoning, etc.)
4 cups chicken broth with salt and spices (see Note)
1 to 2 tablespoons chopped fresh cilantro or parsley (optional)

1. Cut the chicken (or beef) into bite-size chunks and sprinkle with salt and pepper.

2. In a soup pot, sauté the onion in the olive oil over medium heat for about 1 minute. Add the garlic and continue to cook until translucent, about another 2 or 3 minutes.

3. Add the chicken (or beef) and sauté until no longer pink.

4. Add the carrot, celery, and zucchini and sauté until slightly softened, about 5 minutes, stirring often to prevent burning.

5. Add the tomatoes and broth. Bring to a boil, then turn heat down and simmer until all vegetables are tender, about 20 minutes.

6. When ready to serve, add the cilantro or parsley to brighten the flavor.

Note: If you don't have seasoned broth on hand, use plain broth and add ¼ teaspoon salt, ¼ teaspoon black pepper, ⅛ teaspoon cayenne pepper, ¼ teaspoon dried basil, and ¼ teaspoon onion powder.

Time-saving Tip: Make a double batch of soup. Portion the extra soup into 1- or 1½-cup servings and store in snap-lid containers for reheating in the microwave.

Meat Week Variation: Omit the carrot and onion and use 4 celery stalks; substitute 2 cups fresh baby spinach for the zucchini, but add it after the tomatoes and broth.

Vegetarian Option: Substitute 2 packages (about 8 ounces each) of baked tofu, diced, for the chicken. Add the tofu when you add the tomatoes and broth.

MEAT WEEK SOUP

Serves 4

2 tablespoons olive oil

1 garlic clove, minced

1 leek, washed, trimmed, and chopped

½ medium head cauliflower, trimmed of leaves and chopped

1 teaspoon salt

½ teaspoon black pepper

½ teaspoon Herbes de Provence

8 ounces white button mushrooms, sliced

2 chicken breasts, cooked and diced (about 2 cups)

4 cups chicken broth

4 cups fresh spinach

1. In a soup pot, heat the olive oil over medium heat. Add the garlic and leek and sauté until softened, about 3 to 4 minutes.

2. Add the cauliflower, salt, pepper, and Herbes de Provence. Continue to cook for another 5 minutes, stirring often to prevent sticking.

3. Add the mushrooms and cook another minute or so.

4. Add the chicken and chicken broth, bring to a boil, then reduce the heat and cook until the cauliflower begins to soften, about 10 minutes.

5. Add the fresh spinach, a handful at a time, stirring as it wilts.

6. Adjust seasonings and serve.

Maintenance Variation: Add ½ cup diced fresh carrot when you add the cauliflower and/or add a can (14 ounces) of fire-roasted diced tomatoes along with the broth.

Time-saving Tip: Make a double batch of soup to enjoy for another dinner. For lunch, portion into 1 cup servings and store in snap-lid containers that you can reheat in the microwave.

Vegetarian Option: Substitute 2 cups diced baked tofu for the chicken.

BLAT LETTUCE WRAPS

Serves 2

FOR THE FILLING

6 slices bacon, cooked until crisp and drained

1 Hass avocado

Juice of ½ lemon

1 small tomato

Salt

FOR THE DRESSING

¼ cup Basic Blender Mayonnaise (page 272) or commercial
   mayonnaise

Juice of ½ lemon

⅛ teaspoon garlic powder

⅛ teaspoon onion powder

Pinch of salt and pepper

1 cup chopped iceberg lettuce

4 large lettuce leaves (Boston Bibb, red leaf, or similar)

1. Prepare the filling: Crumble the bacon. Halve the avocado and spoon out meat. Dice and douse with the lemon juice, tossing gently to coat the pieces. Dice the tomato and sprinkle with a little salt.

2. Prepare the dressing: In a mixing bowl, combine the mayonnaise, lemon juice, and seasonings and whisk until smooth.

3. Stir the chopped lettuce into the dressing and toss to coat. Add the tomato, bacon, and avocado and gently toss again.

4. Place one-fourth of the salad mixture on the center of each lettuce leaf, fold the sides in, and roll up, burrito style.

Maintenance Variation: Use a low-carb flour tortilla in place of the lettuce leaves.

Vegetarian Option: Substitute turkey or soy bacon for the pork bacon.

CHICKEN CAESAR SALAD LETTUCE WRAPS

Serves 2

If you want to save a step here, substitute pre-cooked rotisserie chicken for the tenders.

4 ounces chicken tenders
Olive oil
Salt and pepper
1 cup chopped romaine lettuce
2 tablespoons Caesar Dressing (page 273)
4 large lettuce leaves (red leaf or Boston Bibb)
4 anchovy fillets (optional)

1. Rub the chicken with a little olive oil, sprinkle with salt and pepper, and grill or broil for 3 or 4 minutes on each side, until cooked through (no pink remaining at the center). Cool and cut into ½-inch dice. You should have about 1 cup cooked chicken.

2. Toss the romaine and chicken with the dressing to coat evenly.

3. Pile one-fourth of the chicken mixture onto the center of each lettuce leaf, top each with an anchovy fillet, and roll up, burrito style.

Maintenance Variation: In Weeks 6 and beyond, you can wrap the salad in a warmed low-carb flour tortilla and/or add shaved curls of Parmesan cheese.

Time-saving Tip: Cook double the chicken tenders, cool, wrap in foil or a zipper-sealed plastic bag and refrigerate for up to 2 days for use in salads or soups.

CHICKEN CLUB SALAD LETTUCE WRAPS

Serves 2

As with the previous recipe, you can opt to save time and use a cooked rotisserie chicken from the deli.

4 ounces grilled chicken tenders
Olive oil
Salt and pepper

FOR THE VINAIGRETTE

1 tablespoon white wine vinegar
¼ teaspoon sea salt
¼ teaspoon minced fresh rosemary
Dash of garlic powder
Dash of onion powder
½ packet Splenda or stevia (optional)
2 tablespoons extra-virgin olive oil

4 strips bacon, cooked until crisp, drained, and crumbled
1 small tomato, diced
1 small ripe avocado, peeled, seeded, and diced
1 tablespoon fresh lime juice
2 thin slices red onion
1 cup chopped romaine lettuce
4 large fresh lettuce leaves (red leaf or Bibb)

1. Prepare the filling: Rub the chicken with a bit of olive oil, sprinkle lightly with salt and pepper, and grill or broil for 3 or 4 minutes on each side, until cooked through (no pink remaining at the center). When cool, cut into ½-inch dice. You should have about 1 cup.

2. Prepare the vinaigrette: Combine the lime juice and seasonings. Let sit for a few minutes, then whisk in the olive oil in a slow stream.

3. Add the chicken, bacon, tomato, avocado, onion, and romaine to the dressing and toss to coat.

4. Center one-fourth of the chicken salad mixture on each of the lettuce leaves and roll up, burrito style.

Maintenance Variation: In Week 6 and beyond, you can also enjoy a serving of this salad wrapped in a warmed low-carb flour tortilla; add 2 tablespoons of shredded Mexican cheese in each wrap, if desired.

Time-saving Tip: Cook double the chicken tenders, cool, wrap in foil or a zipper-sealed plastic bag and refrigerate for up to 2 days for use in soups or salads.

SIMPLE CAESAR SALAD

Serves 4

4 cups chopped romaine lettuce
1 recipe Caesar Dressing (page 273)
8 anchovy fillets (optional)
Parmigiano-Reggiano cheese (optional)

1. Place the romaine in a large bowl. Pour dressing over. Toss to coat all leaves evenly.

2. Serve the salad on individual plates with 2 anchovy fillets criss-crossed on top of each serving, if desired.

3. Using a carrot peeler, shave a few curls from a block of cheese over the top.

Note: Wrap the remaining cheese in a couple of thicknesses of paper towel and an outer layer of waxed paper, and store in the refrigerator for many weeks.

Flavor Variation: Top salad with 1 cup chopped cooked chicken, shrimp, or salmon.

Vegetarian Option: Top salad with cubes of seasoned baked tofu.

CLASSIC COBB SALAD

Serves 4

1 large head iceberg lettuce

8 strips bacon, cooked, drained, and crumbled

1 cup diced cooked chicken

4 hard-boiled eggs, peeled and chopped

1 cup crumbled blue cheese (4 ounces)

1 cup shredded raw carrots

1 cup Creamy Gorgonzola Dressing (page 274)

1. Trim, core, wash, and dry the lettuce thoroughly. Chop coarsely.

2. Divide the lettuce among 4 large bowls.

3. Arrange the bacon, chicken, eggs, blue cheese, and carrots in clusters atop the lettuce.

4. Serve ¼ cup dressing on the side with each serving.

Meat Week Variation: Omit the cheese, add ½ cup extra chicken, and use an olive oil vinaigrette instead.

Vegetarian Option: Substitute 1 cup diced baked tofu for the chicken, substitute 8 to 12 slices soy bacon strips for the pork bacon.

GREEK SALAD

Serves 2

¼ teaspoon minced fresh rosemary

Pinch of dried oregano

Pinch of sea salt

Pinch of black pepper

2 tablespoons red wine vinegar

1 large ripe tomato

1 English cucumber

2 tablespoons olive oil

½ cup feta cheese cubes (optional)

1. In a medium bowl, whisk the herbs, salt, and pepper into the vinegar. Allow the mixture to sit for 5 to 10 minutes to marry the flavors. Stream in the olive oil, whisking to blend.

2. Stem the tomato and trim the cucumber and chop both into ½-inch chunks. (There's no need to peel or seed an English cucumber. If using a cucumber with a wax coating, you may wish to peel and seed it.)

3. Lightly salt the tomato and cucumber, then add them to the bowl with the dressing, and toss to coat well. Let the salad sit for another few minutes at room temperature or, if not serving right away, cover and refrigerate.

4. Just before serving, toss in the feta cubes and gently mix to distribute.

GRILLED CHICKEN SALAD

Serves 2

½ *teaspoon kosher salt*

½ *teaspoon freshly ground black pepper*

¼ *teaspoon paprika*

¼ *teaspoon onion powder*

¼ *teaspoon garlic powder*

1 *tablespoon fresh lemon juice*

1 *teaspoon balsamic vinegar*

1 *teaspoon Dijon mustard*

1 *packet Splenda or stevia*

3 *tablespoons olive oil*

2 *boneless, skinless chicken half breasts or thighs*

4 *cups chopped romaine lettuce*

1. Prepare a charcoal or gas grill. In a small bowl, combine the seasonings, lemon juice, vinegar, mustard, and sweetener. Whisk in the olive oil, blending until emulsified.

2. Rinse the chicken and pat dry with paper towels. Place the chicken in a shallow bowl or pie plate and pour half the dressing over the pieces, turning them to coat well. (Reserve the remaining dressing to dress the salad greens later.) Allow the chicken to marinate in the dressing for 15 minutes. Discard marinade after use.

3. Grill the chicken over medium-high heat for 4 to 5 minutes per side.

4. Meanwhile, toss the salad greens with the reserved dressing to coat lightly, but well. Divide between two plates.

5. Slice the chicken breasts on the diagonal, and lay strips atop the dressed salad greens.

Time-saving Tip: When cooking the chicken, cook a double or even a triple batch. When cooled, slice the extra breasts and store in zipper-sealed plastic bags in the refrigerator for use in soups or salads for up to 2 days.

Maintenance Variation: Add ¼ cup of cheese (feta crumbles, blue cheese crumbles, shredded mozzarella) or a handful of croutons made from low-carb or lite bread, brushed with garlic butter and toasted in a 200° F oven until crisp.

CHICKEN (OR TUNA) SALAD STUFFED TOMATO

Serves 2

1 can (5 to 6 ounces) chicken or tuna, drained
1 celery stalk, finely diced
1 small apple, peeled and finely diced
· *2 green onions, white and green parts, chopped*
2 tablespoons mayonnaise (page 272)
1 tablespoon Dijon mustard
1 tablespoon capers, rinsed and drained
Pinch of salt
Pinch of black pepper
2 ripe medium tomatoes
Olive oil vinaigrette (optional)

1. Place the chicken (or tuna) in a medium bowl and separate with a fork. Add remaining ingredients except the tomatoes, and combine thoroughly.

2. Wash the tomatoes and cut out the stems. Flip them stem end down and slice (from the bottom of the tomato toward the stem end) into 6 wedges as you would a pie. Do not cut all the way through; rather, leave the wedges attached to each other around the hole where the stem was. Spread the wedges apart from the center to make a star or flower with a well in the center.

3. Place a large scoop of chicken (or tuna) salad into this well, mounding it in the center.

4. Drizzle with vinaigrette, if desired. Serve.

Meat Week Variation: Omit the apple and increase the celery to 2 ribs. Add 5 or 6 chopped black or kalamata olives.

Vegetarian Option: Use the Meat Week variation, but for the chicken or tuna, substitute 2 chopped hard-boiled eggs and 3 ounces diced baked tofu.

MEDITERRANEAN CHOPPED SALAD

Serves 4

2 tablespoons red wine vinegar

¾ teaspoon salt

¼ teaspoon black pepper

⅛ teaspoon dried basil

⅛ teaspoon dried oregano

¼ cup olive oil

1 large English cucumber, cut into ½-inch cubes

¼ medium red onion, sliced

2 or 3 red radishes, thinly sliced

1 large tomato, cut into ½-inch cubes

1. In a large bowl, combine the vinegar, salt, pepper, and herbs. Set aside for a few minutes to allow the flavors to combine.

2. Stream in the olive oil slowly, whisking all the while to make the dressing.

3. Add the cucumber, onion, and radishes and toss well to coat. Add the tomatoes and gently toss to coat.

Flavor Variation: Make the salad an entrée by adding diced cooked chicken (or diced tofu for vegetarians).

Maintenance Variation: Add about ½ cup feta cheese cubes along with the tomatoes in the final step.

OLIVE SALAD

Serves 4 to 6

1 *cup pitted brine-cured black olives, sliced*

1 *cup large pimiento-stuffed olives, sliced*

½ *cup extra-virgin olive oil*

2 *tablespoons minced shallot*

2 *tablespoons finely chopped celery*

2 *tablespoons minced fresh flat-leaf parsley*

2 *teaspoons minced garlic*

1½ *teaspoons freshly ground black pepper*

1. Combine all the ingredients in a bowl and mix well.

2. Cover and refrigerate until ready to use. (The salad can be refrigerated for up to 1 week.)

Time-saving Tip: The recipe keeps well in the refrigerator, so make a double or triple batch if you are an olive lover.

SUNNY DAY GARDEN SALAD

Serves 2

½ ripe Hass avocado, seeded, peeled, and diced

Juice of ½ lime

2 cups mixed lettuces

¼ medium jícama, peeled and sliced into matchsticks

½ yellow bell pepper, seeded and sliced into strips

½ cup broccoli slaw

¼ small red onion, thinly sliced

2 tablespoons pine nuts, lightly toasted

3 tablespoons Dijon Vinaigrette (page 276)

1. Douse the avocado with the lime juice and set aside.

2. In a salad bowl, combine the lettuce and vegetables. Add the dressing and toss to coat evenly.

3. Add the avocado and pine nuts, and gently fold them in. Divide the salad evenly between two chilled plates.

Flavor Variation: Add grilled salmon, chicken, shrimp, or even beef for a hearty meal.

Vegetarian Option: Add diced baked tofu.

WARM SESAME AND GINGER SPINACH SALAD

Serves 4

2 tablespoons sesame seeds

6 slices pancetta, coarsely diced

3 tablespoons toasted sesame oil

1 small shallot, finely diced

2 tablespoons rice wine vinegar

1 packet Splenda or stevia (optional)

½ teaspoon salt

¼ teaspoon freshly ground black pepper

¼ teaspoon wasabi paste (from a tube)

1 medium red onion, thinly sliced

6 cups baby spinach leaves

2 tablespoons chopped fresh cilantro

1 packet (about 4 tablespoons) pickled ginger, drained, rinsed, and
    sliced

1. Toast the sesame seeds in a dry skillet over low heat until just turn-ing golden; set aside.

2. In a skillet, fry the pancetta in the sesame oil over medium-high heat until crisp, about 3 to 5 minutes. Remove with a slotted spoon and drain on paper towels. Leave the oil in the skillet, but turn the heat off or down to the lowest simmer, depending on how long it will be before you eat the salad.

3. In a small heatproof bowl, combine the shallot, vinegar, sweetener (if using), salt, pepper, and wasabi paste and whisk to combine.

4. Add the onion slices to the vinegar mixture and allow to marinate for at least 10 minutes to remove some of their bite. Remove the onion from the vinegar with a slotted spoon and set aside.

5. When ready to assemble (and eat) the salad, place the fresh spinach, pancetta, cilantro, pickled ginger, and onion in a large salad bowl and have ready.

6. Return the skillet to medium-high heat to get the oil hot, but not smoking. Turn off the heat and drizzle the hot oil into the vinegar mixture, whisking all the while. Immediately pour the hot dressing over the spinach salad and toss quickly to coat evenly and slightly wilt the leaves.

7. Sprinkle on the toasted sesame seeds and give another quick toss to distribute them. Serve.

Vegetarian Option: Substitute 6 slices of soy bacon strips for the pancetta.

BEEF, PORK, AND LAMB

ANTIPASTO LUNCH PLATE

Serves 1

1 to 2 ounces hard salami slices

1 to 2 ounces turkey or chicken slices

1 hard-boiled egg, peeled and sliced

4 to 6 marinated green beans

4 to 6 large olives

3 to 4 whole pepperoncini (hot or mild)

Arrange all the items on a plate and enjoy.

Flavor Variation: For an antipasto salad, scatter the items on a bed of arugula, lightly dressed with Dijon Vinaigrette (page 276).

Maintenance Variation: Add 1 or 2 ounces of Italian cheeses, such as pecorino or fontina, to the plate.

Vegetarian Option: Omit the salami and turkey and substitute slices of baked tofu or smoked trout or salmon.

BEEF TENDERLOIN AND ASPARAGUS ROLL-UPS

Serves 2 (or 1 hearty appetite)

½ *pound roasted beef tenderloin or deli roast beef, very thinly sliced*
16 *to* 20 *marinated asparagus spears*
Dijon mustard

1. Lay the beef slices on a flat surface and spread each with about ¼ teaspoon of Dijon mustard.

2. Place 1 or 2 marinated asparagus spears across the slice near the front edge.

3. Roll the slice over the asparagus and keep rolling to the far edge. Secure with a toothpick if needed.

Flavor Variation: Substitute marinated green beans or coarsely chopped Giardiniera (jarred hot marinated vegetables, available in the pickle aisle of most grocery stores).

GARLIC-RUBBED BEEF TENDERLOIN

Serves 4

3 garlic cloves

1 teaspoon coarse salt

1 tablespoon olive oil

1 to 1½ pounds beef tenderloin

1 tablespoon minced fresh rosemary

1 tablespoon minced fresh sage

1 teaspoon black pepper

3 tablespoons melted butter (optional)

1. Preheat the oven to 500° F.

2. Mince the garlic and sprinkle on the salt. With the flat blade of your knife, work the salt and garlic into a paste, then incorporate the olive oil.

3. Rub the garlic paste over the meat. Evenly scatter the herbs and pepper over the surface.

4. Place the tenderloin into a roasting pan and roast for about 5 minutes in the very hot oven.

5. Turn the oven off, leave the door closed, and allow roast to finish cooking for the next 4 hours as the oven slowly cools. Do not open the oven door for 4 hours.

6. Slice the tenderloin to serve at room temperature or reheat the slices gently in melted butter in a skillet to serve warm.

Flavor Variation: Substitute pork tenderloin, but roast for 7 to 10 minutes before proceeding to step 5 and turning the oven off.

ROAST PORK AND VEGGIE STIR-FRY

Makes 4 servings

8 ounces cooked Garlic-Rubbed Pork Tenderloin (page 213 variation)

1 teaspoon Chinese Five Spice powder

2 tablespoons sesame or peanut oil

1 garlic clove, peeled

1 cup cabbage slaw mix

1 cup broccoli slaw mix

¼ teaspoon red chile paste (optional)

2 tablespoons soy sauce

1. Slice the cooked tenderloin into thin pieces about 1 inch long. Sprinkle with Chinese Five Spice powder and set aside.

2. Heat oil in a skillet or wok over high heat until almost smoking.

3. Add the garlic clove and the slaw mixtures and stir-fry for 2 to 3 minutes, until beginning to get tender.

4. Add the sliced pork, chile paste, and soy sauce and continue to stir-fry until the meat is heated through.

5. Serve hot over Fried Cauli-Rice (page 258).

Vegetarian Option: Substitute seasoned baked tofu (diced) for the pork.

GRILLED HERB-CRUSTED LAMB T-BONES

Serves 2

1 tablespoon chopped fresh thyme, or ½ teaspoon dried

1 tablespoon chopped fresh rosemary, or ½ teaspoon dried

1 tablespoon chopped fresh mint

2 garlic cloves, minced finely

1 teaspoon coarse salt

1 teaspoon black pepper

4 to 6 loin lamb chops

2 tablespoons olive oil

Minted Vinegar (page 277)

1. In a shallow bowl or pie plate thoroughly combine all the herbs and seasonings.

2. Brush both sides of each chop with olive oil and lay first one side then the other onto the herb mixture. Press lightly to encourage the meat to pick up the herb coating.

3. Place the coated chops into a zipper-sealed plastic bag or covered container and let marinate for at least 30 minutes at room temperature. (You can marinate overnight in the refrigerator, but if you do, omit the salt from the herb mixture and add it by sprinkling on both sides just before grilling.)

4. Lightly oil a grill pan or outdoor grill grate and then preheat to medium-high heat.

5. Grill the chops about 4 minutes per side for medium-rare. Serve with Minted Vinegar.

ROSEMARY AND MINT RACK OF LAMB

Serves 2

1 rack of lamb (6 to 8 bones)

1 teaspoon sea salt

½ teaspoon freshly ground black pepper

2 tablespoons unsalted butter

1 tablespoon chopped fresh mint

1 teaspoon chopped fresh rosemary

1 clove garlic, finely chopped

1 tablespoon freshly grated parmesan cheese

1. Preheat the oven to 450° F.

2. Sprinkle the lamb rack on both sides with the salt and pepper.

3. In a microwave-safe bowl, melt the butter on high for 30 to 40 seconds. Stir in the chopped herbs, garlic, and cheese. Set aside.

4. On the stovetop, heat a dry oven-proof skillet over high heat. When skillet is hot, sear the rack bone tips up for 2 minutes, then turn rack and sear bone tips down for 1 minute.

5. Brush the herbed butter mixture over both sides of the rack.

6. Place the skillet containing the rack into the oven and roast for 15 minutes.

7. Remove the skillet from the oven and allow the rack to rest for 10 minutes before carving into individual chops.

GRILLED SPICE-RUBBED FLANK STEAK

Serves 4

2 tablespoons soy sauce
1½ to 2 pounds flank steak
1 tablespoon olive oil

FOR THE SPICE RUB

1½ tablespoons paprika
1 tablespoon chili powder
1 teaspoon garlic powder
1 teaspoon onion powder
1 teaspoon ground cumin
1 teaspoon black pepper
½ teaspoon dry mustard
¼ teaspoon cayenne pepper (optional)

1. Sprinkle the soy sauce over both sides of the meat and allow to sit for 5 minutes. Rub both sides of the flank steak with olive oil.

2. Meanwhile, in a zipper-sealed plastic bag combine the ingredients for the spice rub. Seal and shake to mix well. Sprinkle half the spice rub on one side of the steak and lightly rub to distribute across the surface. Repeat with the remaining half of the rub on the other side. Place the meat in a large zipper-sealed plastic bag, seal, and let marinate at room temperature for at least 30 minutes.

3. Clean and oil the grill grates and preheat the grill (or a grill pan) to medium-high. You will need a cool place on the grill (away from the heat source); this could be a shelf or an area of the grill under which the burner is not turned on or there is no charcoal underneath. (If this isn't possible, finish the steak in a 350° F oven.)

4. Sear the steak on the hot grill for 1 minute. Turn it a quarter-turn on the same side and sear for another minute to make a cross-hatch of grill marks. Flip the steak over and repeat to sear and cross-hatch on the

other side. Remove the steak to the cooler area of the grill, close cover, and cook for an additional 10 minutes for medium-rare.

5. Allow the meat to rest at least 5 minutes, then slice it against the grain into approximately ¼-inch slices.

Time-saving Tip: Prepare two flank steaks at once. Serve one and, when cooled, refrigerate the other for up to 3 days in a clean zipper-sealed plastic bag for snacking, lunches, or to gently reheat for dinner.

GYRO BURGERS

Serves 4

You'll need at least 30 minutes (but up to a day) in advance to make the tzatziki sauce.

4 fresh lamb and mint sausages, about polish dog size, 7 inches long (see Note)

FOR THE TZATZIKI SAUCE

½ medium cucumber
8 to 10 large fresh mint leaves
1 garlic clove, crushed
½ cup plain yogurt (preferably Greek)
1 tablespoon red wine vinegar, or more to taste
½ teaspoon coarse sea salt, or more to taste
¼ teaspoon freshly ground black pepper, or more to taste
¼ teaspoon onion powder
1 ounce lemon juice

FOR THE CONDIMENT SALAD

1 small white or yellow onion
Juice of ½ lemon
1 medium tomato
Coarse sea salt and freshly ground pepper to taste
½ medium cucumber
1 tablespoon red wine vinegar
2 tablespoons extra-virgin olive oil (Greek if you've got it)

1. To make the tzatziki sauce: Peel and seed the cucumber half. Cut into chunks and put into the workbowl of a food processor.

2. Add the mint leaves, garlic, yogurt, vinegar, salt, pepper, onion powder, and lemon juice. Blend until smooth. Taste and adjust season-

ings, adding a bit more salt, pepper, and/or vinegar to achieve a piquant flavor.

3. Pour into a container, cover tightly, and refrigerate for 30 minutes or longer to develop the flavors.

1. To make the condiment salad: Peel and thinly slice the onion, and place it in a small bowl; cover with water and a splash of lemon juice and let it soak a few minutes to take away the "bite."

2. Seed and dice the tomato and the other cucumber half; place them in a bowl and sprinkle with a little sea salt (to taste) and pepper.

3. Add the vinegar and olive oil and toss gently to coat.

4. Just before serving, add the onion and toss again to combine.

When ready to grill or griddle the meat

1. Prepare a charcoal grill or preheat a gas grill.

2. Split the sausage casings lengthwise and peel away from the meat; discard casings. Press the link into a flat, thin patty no more than ½-inch thick.

3. Grill the thin patties for 2½ to 3 minutes per side; remove from the grill to a plate and let rest for a few minutes.

4. Slice each patty in half lengthwise before serving. Top each burger with a tablespoon or two of tzatziki sauce and top with a mound of condiment salad and a bit more sauce.

Maintenance Variation: Wrap the gyro burger in a warm low-carb tortilla.

Vegetarian Option: Make the burgers using ground turkey or chicken or substitute meatless burgers. The taste won't be quite the same as a gyro, but the tzatziki sauce is still yummy.

Note: If you can't find fresh lamb sausages at your butcher counter, use 1 pound ground lamb and add 2 tablespoons chopped fresh mint, 1 clove garlic, minced, ¼ teaspoon salt, ¼ teaspoon black pepper, ¼ teaspoon onion powder and mix thoroughly.

INSIDE OUT TRIPLE-DECKER HAM SANDWICH

Serves 1

3 slices baked ham, about ¼-inch thick
Basic Blender Mayonnaise (page 272)
Mustard of choice
1 large fresh lettuce leaf
2 slices ripe tomato
Salt and pepper

1. Lay the ham slices on a flat surface and spread liberally on one side with mayonnaise, mustard, or both.

2. Tear the lettuce leaf in half. Place one half of the leaf on a slice of ham, top with a slice of tomato, and sprinkle with salt and pepper.

3. Place a second slice of ham atop the stack you've begun, add the other half of the lettuce leaf, and another tomato slice and sprinkle again with salt and pepper.

4. Top with the remaining ham slice.

Time-saving Tip: This dish is a great use for leftover ham after the holidays or any time.

LAMB AND RED PEPPER KEBABS

Serves 2

You can easily multiply these ingredients for more kebabs.

1 *large red bell pepper*
1 *large sweet onion*

FOR THE MARINADE

¼ *cup olive oil*
2 *tablespoons red wine vinegar*
1 *tablespoon chopped fresh mint leaves*
1 *garlic clove, crushed*
2 *tablespoons soy sauce*
½ *teaspoon black pepper*

1 *pound boneless lamb chunks for stew*

1. Remove the stem and seeds from the pepper and cut into quarters, then cut the quarters in half to make 8 chunks.

2. Cut the onion into 8 wedges.

3. In a large zipper-sealed plastic bag, mix the ingredients for the marinade, add the lamb chunks and vegetables and seal tightly. Allow to marinate for 30 minutes at room temperature or overnight in the refrigerator.

4. Preheat a charcoal grill, grill pan, or broiler. Oil the grate well while still cold. Bring meat and vegetables to room temperature. If using bamboo skewers, soak them in water for at least 20 minutes before using to prevent burning.

5. Thread the meat onto a couple of the skewers, and the vegetables separately onto the other skewers, allowing for differing cooking times of these items.

6. Place the onion skewers on the grill first and cook for 1 to 2 minutes on each side. Add the meat skewers and cook for 4 minutes; turn

both meat and onion skewers to cook evenly. Add the pepper skewers and cook for 4 minutes.

7. Remove the meat and allow to rest while the onion and pepper skewers finish cooking, another few minutes.

8. Divide the meat, onion, and pepper between the plates and serve.

MEAT WEEK CHILI

Serves 4 to 6

2 tablespoons chili powder

1 teaspoon ground cumin

1 teaspoon sea salt

1 teaspoon ground black pepper

¼ teaspoon cayenne pepper, or to taste (optional)

1½ pounds ground sirloin

2 tablespoons coconut oil or olive oil

1 garlic clove, crushed

¼ medium onion, grated

¼ small green bell pepper, seeded and diced

½ cup chopped white mushrooms

1 can (about 14 ounces) diced roasted tomatoes

4 cups beef broth

1. Mix the seasonings in a small bowl.

2. Sprinkle half of the seasoning mixture over the ground sirloin, knead through, and let sit at room temperature for at least 30 minutes to flavor the beef.

3. In a large skillet or soup pot, heat the oil over medium heat. Add the garlic, onion, and bell pepper and sauté until bell pepper softens slightly and the onion is translucent, about 3 to 5 minutes.

4. Add the mushroom pieces and sauté until they begin to brown, then add the remaining seasoning mix and stir to mix thoroughly.

5. Add the ground sirloin and brown well, then add the tomatoes and broth, and stir to combine. Reduce the heat and simmer, uncovered, for at least 30 minutes, reducing the liquid by half.

6. Serve immediately or cool, cover, and refrigerate for up to 4 days.

Maintenance Variation: Increase the bell pepper to ½ pepper and the onion to ½ an onion, and add 1 grated small carrot in step 3. To finish

the dish, add a handful of shredded Mexican-blend cheese and a sprinkling of chopped green onions.

Time-saving Tip: Make a double batch and portion 1-cup or 1½-cup
individual servings into snap-lid containers for reheating in the
microwave for lunches, dinners, or snacks. Store the individual containers for up to 3 days in the refrigerator or freeze them for up to a
month. Thaw frozen chili overnight in the refrigerator for best results
before reheating.

Vegetarian/No-Beef Options: Replace the beef broth with vegetable or
mushroom broth and the sirloin with ground turkey or 1 pound equivalent of soy-based TVP or 4 to 6 crumbled veggie burger patties.

PORK TENDERLOIN ROAST

Serves 4 to 6

1 teaspoon kosher salt

1 teaspoon coarsely ground black pepper

1 teaspoon garlic powder

2 to 2½ pounds boneless pork tenderloin

1 tablespoon unsalted butter (optional)

1. Preheat the oven to 500° F.

2. Combine the salt, pepper, and garlic powder and mix well.

3. Sprinkle the seasoning mixture evenly over the meat. Place the meat in a roasting pan, and roast for 5 to 7 minutes.

4. Turn the oven off, but do not open the door for at least 3 hours. The meat will continue to cook as the oven temperature slowly drops.

5. Slice into ½-inch medallions. Rewarm or serve cold (in wraps or on salads). To serve warm, melt 1 tablespoon butter in a skillet over medium heat and gently warm the slices.

Flavor Variation: Substitute beef tenderloin, but for medium-rare, turn the oven off immediately upon putting in the tenderloin; for medium, roast 5 minutes before turning oven off.

STUFFED BUFFALO (OR BEEF) BURGERS

Serves 4

1 pound ground buffalo (or lean beef)

1 tablespoon soy sauce

½ teaspoon garlic powder

½ teaspoon freshly ground black pepper

1 can (about 4 ounces) mild diced green chile

4 tablespoons shredded Mexican cheese blend

1. Preheat gas or charcoal grill to medium-hot.

2. In a medium bowl, mix the ground meat with the soy sauce, garlic, and black pepper until evenly distributed.

3. Divide mixture roughly into 4 equal portions, then divide each portion in half to make 8 portions of meat. Pat each of these portions into a patty about ¼-inch thick.

4. Put about 1 tablespoon of diced chile and 1 tablespoon shredded cheese into the center of 4 of the patties. Top each patty with another patty and press the edges together all around to make a tight seal. Then gently reshape the patties to make them smooth again. You will have 4 thick, stuffed burger patties.

5. Grill or broil the burgers over medium-high heat for 4 to 5 minutes per side or to desired level of doneness. (Buffalo is quite lean, so watch carefully—overcooking will make it tough.)

Meat Week Variation: Omit the cheese.

TRIPLE-THREAT MEATLOAF

Serves 4

2 tablespoons olive oil

½ medium yellow onion

¼ yellow bell pepper, seeded and diced

¼ green bell pepper, seeded and diced

¼ red bell pepper, seeded and diced

2 large eggs

¼ cup heavy cream

1 tablespoon Worcestershire sauce

1 teaspoon sea salt

½ teaspoon black pepper

½ teaspoon paprika

¼ teaspoon garlic powder

⅛ teaspoon cayenne pepper (optional)

½ pound ground sirloin

½ pound ground pork

½ pound ground lamb

1. Heat the olive oil in a skillet over medium heat; add the onion and sauté until translucent. Add the bell peppers and continue to cook, stirring occasionally, until they begin to soften, about 3 minutes. Allow to cool slightly.

2. In a large mixing bowl, beat the eggs well. Add the cream, onion, and bell peppers, and then all the seasonings, and stir to combine.

3. Add the ground meats and knead to mix evenly.

4. Lightly oil a microwave-safe loaf pan and press the meat mixture into the pan to form a loaf. Cover with a paper towel to prevent splatters. Microwave on full power for 15 minutes, turning pan once if microwave is not equipped with a carousel. Reduce power to 80 percent and continue to cook for another 10 to 12 minutes, depending on wattage of your oven—lesser power ovens may take longer. (You

can also bake the meatloaf in a conventional oven at 350° F for
1 hour.)

Time-saving Tip: Bake two loaves, sequentially, in the microwave
to have extra servings for subsequent meals, such as for sandwiches,
protein-style. (In a conventional oven, two meatloaves cook as quickly
as one.)

CHICKEN AND POULTRY

BEER-CAN CHICKEN

Serves 4

FOR THE SPICE RUB

1 tablespoon paprika

1 teaspoon garlic powder

1 teaspoon onion powder

1 teaspoon sea salt

½ teaspoon dry mustard

½ teaspoon ground cumin

½ teaspoon freshly ground black pepper

¼ teaspoon cayenne pepper

1 can light beer

1 to 2 tablespoons olive oil

1 broiler-fryer chicken, 2 to 3 pounds

1. Preheat a covered charcoal or gas grill to medium-hot.

2. In a bowl or zipper-sealed plastic bag, combine the ingredients for the spice rub.

3. Pop the top on the beer, pour half into a glass (to drink, if you like) and rub the can with olive oil, being careful not to spill remaining beer in can.

4. Rub the chicken all over, including the cavity, with olive oil. Sprinkle 1 teaspoon of the spice rub into the cavity, then rub the remainder over the chicken.

5. Place a 12-inch square of aluminum foil on the grill where the chicken will go to prevent flare-ups. Insert the beer can into the chicken

cavity, open top first. Set the chicken and can onto the aluminum foil square, balancing the chicken on the can and its legs.

6. Close the grill lid and grill for 45 minutes to 1 hour. Check for doneness with an instant-read meat thermometer inserted into the thickest portion of the thigh, away from bone. When the temperature reaches 160° F, remove the chicken and let rest for approximately 10 minutes before carving. (Take care removing the chicken from the beer can; use oven mitts or a thick wad of paper towels in each hand.)

Time-saver Tip: Grill 2 or even 3 chickens at once if they will fit in your grill with the lid closed. Allow the extra chickens to cool and store them, whole or cut into pieces, in a zipper-sealed plastic bag for dinners or lunches for several days, or use the meat to make chicken salads or soups.

BUFFALO CHICKEN WINGS

Serves 4

FOR THE BUFFALO SAUCE

½ cup water
¼ cup olive oil
¼ cup red wine vinegar
2 tablespoons tomato paste
1 tablespoon chili powder
¼ teaspoon cayenne pepper or Tabasco sauce, or to taste

2 pounds chicken wings
Coarse salt and black pepper

1. Make the sauce in advance: Combine the ingredients in a saucepan over medium-high heat, stirring occasionally, and bring to a boil. Boil for 5 minutes, remove from the heat, and set aside.

2. Preheat the oven to 400° F and heat a stovetop grill pan over medium-high heat.

3. Wash the wings and pat dry. Remove the tips from the wings with a heavy knife or poultry shears and sever the wing at the joint to make 2 pieces. Sprinkle the wings with salt and pepper, arrange in the grill pan, and cook for about 2 minutes on each side.

4. Remove the wings from the pan and arrange on an oiled baking sheet. Roast in the oven for 20 to 30 minutes.

5. Reduce the oven to 350° F, flip the wings over, and roast for another 20 to 30 minutes.

6. Reduce the oven temperature to 200° F, flip the wings again, and cook for another 20 to 30 minutes. Turn oven off.

7. Remove the wings from the oven and immediately dip each wing into the sauce and arrange on a serving platter. (You can keep the wings warm for up to 30 minutes, covered with foil, in the cooling oven.)

CHICKEN MUSHROOM PACKETS

Serves 4

Thin slices of chicken breast are available at most markets. If you cannot find them, then pound a boneless, skinless chicken breast between sheets of waxed paper. This recipe originally appeared in our book *The Low Carb CookwoRx Cookbook* (Wiley, 2005).

*1 cup dried wild mushrooms, rehydrated, or 1 can (8 ounces) sliced
    mushrooms*
1 teaspoon salt
1 teaspoon ground black pepper
1 teaspoon rubbed sage
4 thin slices boneless, skinless breast (about 3/8 inch thick)
2 tablespoons olive oil, or more as needed
2 tablespoons unsalted butter, softened
1 tablespoon ThickenThin not/Starch, or 2 teaspoons xanthan gum
1/2 cup heavy cream

1. If using dried mushrooms, rehydrate in warm water for about 15 minutes until plump.

2. Tear four 12-inch squares of aluminum foil and brush one side of each with a bit of olive oil.

3. Preheat the oven to 350° F.

4. In a small bowl, mix 1/2 teaspoon each of the salt, pepper, and sage.

5. Rinse the chicken slices and pat dry with paper towels. Rub the slices all over with about a teaspoon of olive oil and sprinkle with half the seasoning mix evenly on both sides. Place a fillet in the center of each piece of foil.

6. In a small bowl, cream together the butter, thickener, and remaining seasoning mix, then incorporate the cream to make a smooth, thick sauce.

7. Drain the mushrooms; if large, chop coarsely. Fold the mushrooms into the cream mixture and divide mixture evenly among the chicken pieces.

8. Drizzle a bit more olive oil over each chicken slice and then make loose packets of each foil square. Bring the opposite corners to the center and crimp the foil at the 4 seams. (Packets can be refrigerated at this point for up to 24 hours. Bring to room temperature before cooking.)

9. Place the packets on a baking sheet and bake for about 30 minutes, or until chicken is fully cooked (ideally to an internal temperature of 165° F). Serve immediately.

CHICKEN WITH 40 CLOVES OF GARLIC

Serves 4

Certainly you can use fewer cloves of garlic, but it won't be the same dish. Because the cloves are roasted and kept whole, the dish is not nearly as garlicky as you might imagine.

4 chicken breast halves, skin on

4 chicken thighs (no drumsticks), skin on

½ cup plus 2 tablespoons olive oil

Salt, pepper, and paprika

4 sprigs fresh thyme, or ½ teaspoon dried

2 sprigs fresh rosemary, or ½ teaspoon dried

40 cloves garlic, peeled but left whole

1. Preheat the oven to 350° F.

2. Rub the chicken with 2 tablespoons of olive oil and sprinkle lightly with salt, pepper, and paprika.

3. Brown the chicken in a large, wide ovenproof skillet or roasting pan over high heat turning as needed, about 4 minutes per side.

4. Remove from the heat, add the remaining olive oil and the rosemary and thyme sprigs, and the 40 cloves of garlic. Cover and bake for 1½ hours.

GOURMET NUTTY BIRD BURGERS

Serves 4

1 pound ground turkey

⅓ cup pine nuts

2 green onions, green and white parts chopped

2 tablespoons chopped fresh parsley

1 teaspoon poultry seasoning

½ teaspoon sea salt

½ teaspoon black pepper

¼ teaspoon garlic powder

¼ teaspoon onion powder

2 tablespoons olive oil

8 large lettuce leaves

4 tablespoons Cranberry-Orange Relish (page 279)

Basic Blender Mayonnaise (page 272; optional)

1. In a bowl, combine the ground turkey, pine nuts, green onions, parsley, seasonings, and 1 tablespoon olive oil. Mix well and form mixture into 4 patties.

2. Heat the remaining tablespoon olive oil in a large skillet over medium-high heat. Fry the turkey burgers about 4 minutes per side, then remove to paper towels to drain.

3. Place each burger onto a large crunchy lettuce leaf, top with 1 tablespoon Cranberry-Orange Relish, add a bit of mayonnaise if desired, top with a second lettuce leaf, and serve.

Maintenance Variation: Wrap the turkey burgers in a low-carb flour tortilla or "lite" hamburger bun. Add a slice of cheese during the last few minutes of cooking, for a turkey cheeseburger.

Vegetarian Option: Substitute TVP burger replacer, prepared according to package instructions.

Time-saving Tip: Triple the recipe to make a dozen burgers at once.

Wrap individual uncooked burgers in zipper-sealed plastic bags or plastic wrap and freeze for up to a month. For best texture and flavor, thaw in the refrigerator overnight before cooking. Or, wrap individual cooked burgers in zipper-sealed plastic bags and store in the refrigerator for lunches or dinners; they will keep for several days.

HERB-ROASTED CHICKEN

Serves 4

½ cup kosher salt

4 cups water

1 broiler-fryer chicken, 3 pounds

4 tablespoons (½ stick) unsalted butter, softened

1 teaspoon salt

¼ teaspoon black pepper

1 garlic clove

1 teaspoon minced fresh rosemary, or ½ teaspoon dried

1 teaspoon minced fresh chives, or ½ teaspoon dried

1 teaspoon minced fresh flat-leaf parsley, or ½ teaspoon dried

Olive oil, for oiling roasting rack

1. In a large bowl or gallon zipper-sealed plastic bag, dissolve the salt in the water and add the chicken. Cover or seal and brine the chicken overnight in the refrigerator. The next day, rinse the chicken and pat dry with paper towels.

2. Preheat the oven to 375° F.

3. In a small bowl, combine the butter with the salt, pepper, garlic, and herbs. Knead until well combined.

4. With the point of a sharp knife, loosen the skin over the breasts at the neck end of the chicken and, with your fingers, create a pocket over each breast between the skin and the meat. Stuff about 1 tablespoon of the herb butter into each pocket.

5. Rub another 1 tablespoon of the herb butter over the skin of the chicken. Reserve the last tablespoon of herb butter for basting the roasted chicken.

6. Place the chicken on an oiled roasting rack, breast side down, and roast for 20 minutes. Turn the bird on its left side and roast for another 10 minutes, then on its right side and roast another 10 minutes.

7. Melt the remaining herb butter in the microwave.

8. Turn the bird breast side up, brush with the melted herb butter, and roast a final 20 minutes, or until the juices run clear (or thigh temperature reaches 165° F).

LEMON CHICKEN

Serves 4 to 6

Boneless breasts work just as well in this classic recipe.

⅓ cup olive oil

3 pounds chicken thighs, washed and patted dry

Salt and pepper to taste

2 large lemons, cut into wedges

1 medium onion, halved and cut into thick slices

3 garlic cloves, minced

1 tablespoon minced fresh thyme, or 1 teaspoon dried

1 tablespoon minced fresh marjoram, or 1 teaspoon dried

1 tablespoon minced fresh parsley, or 1 teaspoon dried

1 teaspoon coarsely ground black pepper

1. Lightly oil a roasting pan with a bit of the olive oil and arrange the chicken thighs in it in a single layer. Sprinkle the chicken with salt and pepper and squeeze on the lemon juice. Lay the spent lemon wedges on top of the chicken.

2. In a separate bowl, combine the onion, garlic, herbs, black pepper, and remaining olive oil and pour the mixture over the chicken thighs.

3. Cover and marinate in the refrigerator for at least 3 hours or as long as overnight.

4. When ready to bake, remove chicken from refrigerator and preheat the oven to 350° F.

5. Bake the chicken thighs, uncovered, for 1 hour, or to an internal temperature of 165° F.

Time-saving Tip: Bake a double batch of thighs. Place the cooled cooked chicken into zipper-sealed plastic bags and store in the refrigerator to enjoy for lunches and dinners, or to use in salads or soup for several days.

MACADAMIA-CRUSTED CHICKEN PAILLARD

Serves 4

If you have time, brine the chicken breasts overnight in a solution of ¼ cup kosher salt and 1 quart water. If you do, omit the salt for the coating mixture. When ready to cook, rinse the breasts and pat dry.

1 cup macadamia nuts

1 large egg, lightly beaten

¼ cup half-and-half

½ teaspoon salt

½ teaspoon black pepper

¼ teaspoon paprika

¼ teaspoon garlic powder

4 boneless and skinless chicken breast halves

2 tablespoons butter

2 tablespoons olive oil

1. Place the macadamia nuts into the workbowl of a food processor and pulse to crush them into small pieces, but not to a fine powder. Spread them in a shallow bowl or pie pan.

2. In another shallow bowl or pie pan, mix the beaten egg, half-and-half, salt, pepper, paprika, and garlic powder.

3. Place breasts between two pieces of waxed paper or plastic wrap and pound until flat.

4. Heat the butter and olive oil in a large, wide skillet over medium-high heat. Dip the chicken breasts in the egg mixture to coat both sides, then dredge in the macadamia nuts to coat both sides.

5. Lay the breasts in the hot skillet, and sauté about 3 to 4 minutes per side, or until the juices run clear. (A meat thermometer reading of 165° F assures safety for chicken.)

THAI CHICKEN LETTUCE WRAPS

Serves 2

4 boneless, skinless chicken thighs

¼ cup soy sauce

Juice of 1 lime

1 garlic clove, crushed

1 tablespoon grated fresh ginger

¼ teaspoon black pepper

¼ teaspoon Thai red chile paste, or a pinch of cayenne

2 tablespoons light sesame oil

1 teaspoon toasted sesame oil

1 can (about 4 ounces) sliced water chestnuts, drained

2 tablespoons toasted sesame seeds

6 large butter lettuce leaves, washed and patted dry

2 green onions, green and white parts chopped

6 tablespoons broccoli (or other) sprouts

6 large sprigs cilantro

1. Dice the chicken into ½-inch pieces and place into a zipper-sealed plastic bag or covered bowl with the soy sauce, lime juice, garlic, ginger, black pepper, and chile paste. Seal and marinate for at least 1 hour (or as long as overnight) in the refrigerator.

2. Heat the sesame oils in a wok or large skillet over medium-high heat.

3. Dice the water chestnuts. Have the sesame seeds, lettuce leaves, green onions, sprouts, and cilantro ready.

4. When the oil is hot, stir-fry the chicken for 2 or 3 minutes. Add the water chestnuts, green onions, and sesame seeds, and continue stir-frying another 2 or 3 minutes, until chicken is cooked.

5. To assemble the wraps, place one lettuce leaf on a plate, spoon one-sixth of the chicken mixture into the center, then add a tablespoon of broccoli sprouts and a sprig of cilantro. Fold the sides in toward the

middle and roll up burrito style. Repeat with the remaining leaves, for 6 wraps.

Flavor Variations: For Thai beef wraps, substitute 4 ounces diced tenderloin or lean beef for the chicken. For Thai shrimp wraps, substitute tiny (cocktail size) canned shrimp. Marinate as directed in recipe, but wait to add the shrimp along with the green onions and water chestnuts, and just heat through.

FISH AND SEAFOOD

AHI TUNA TARTARE

Serves 2

1 teaspoon rice wine vinegar

½ teaspoon balsamic vinegar

1 teaspoon soy sauce

¼ teaspoon wasabi paste

½ teaspoon grated fresh ginger, or ¼ teaspoon dried

½ packet Splenda or stevia, or other noncaloric sweetener of your choice

4 ounces fresh sashimi-grade ahi (yellowfin) tuna

1½ tablespoons light sesame oil

1 teaspoon roasted sesame oil

1 teaspoon toasted sesame seeds

1 small bunch watercress, washed, trimmed, and dried

1 tablespoon pickled ginger (optional)

1. In a small bowl, whisk together the vinegars, soy sauce, wasabi, ginger, and Splenda. Let sit for 10 or 15 minutes to marry the flavors and infuse the liquid with the ginger.

2. Dice the tuna into ½-inch pieces and place into a bowl large enough to toss them with dressing. (Placing the ahi, wrapped in plastic, in the freezer for about 15 minutes beforehand will make it firmer and easier to cut.)

3. Drizzle the oils into the vinegars slowly while whisking to blend well. Pour all but 1 teaspoon of the dressing over the diced tuna and toss gently to coat evenly.

4. Divide mixture, centering each serving on a chilled plate. Drizzle a bit of the reserved dressing onto each plate and sprinkle on the sesame seeds. Finish each plate with half of the watercress and a side of pickled ginger, if desired.

BAKED SALSA SNAPPER

Serves 4

4 tablespoons olive oil

4 red snapper fillets (4 to 5 ounces each)

Pinch of sea salt

Pinch of black pepper

1 can (14 ounces) diced tomatoes with green chiles, drained

¼ cup capers, drained

2 garlic cloves, thinly sliced

Juice and zest of 1 lime

¼ teaspoon ground cumin

½ teaspoon ground chile

⅛ teaspoon garlic powder

2 green onions, green and white parts chopped

2 tablespoons chopped fresh cilantro

1. Preheat the oven to 425° F. Use a bit of the oil to coat a baking pan large enough to accommodate the fillets without crowding.

2. Season the fish on both sides with salt and pepper and lay them side by side in the dish.

3. In a separate bowl, combine the remaining olive oil and the tomatoes, capers, garlic, lime juice and zest, and seasoning.

4. Spoon the tomato mixture onto the fish and bake for about 10 minutes, or until the fish is lightly golden and flaky.

5. Scatter the green onions and cilantro over the top and serve.

Variation: Substitute trout fillets, orange roughy, or any other mild white fish for the snapper.

CIOPPINO (FISHERMAN'S STEW)

Serves 4

2 tablespoons olive oil

1 small yellow onion, chopped

½ green bell pepper, seeded and chopped

2 sun-dried tomatoes packed in oil, drained and chopped

1 bottle (8 ounces) clam juice

1 can (14 ounces) fire-roasted diced tomatoes with juice

2 garlic cloves, minced

1 teaspoon fresh thyme leaves

1 teaspoon minced fresh rosemary

1 tablespoon minced fresh basil

1 bay leaf

½ cup dry red wine

4 cups fish or chicken stock

1 pound firm, white fish fillets, cut into chunks

½ pound sea scallops, cut into chunks if large

½ teaspoon coarse salt

½ teaspoon freshly ground black pepper

1 teaspoon fennel seeds, crushed

4 tablespoons freshly grated Parmesan cheese

1 tablespoon chopped fresh flat-leaf parsley or cilantro

1. Heat the olive oil in a large saucepan or soup pot and sauté the onion and bell pepper until soft, about 3 to 4 minutes.

2. Meanwhile, in a blender, puree the sun-dried tomatoes with the clam juice until smooth. Add the tomato-clam puree to the pot along with the diced tomatoes, garlic, herbs, wine, and stock. Simmer for about 20 minutes.

3. Meanwhile, season the fish and scallops with salt, pepper, and fennel seeds, and set aside.

4. Add the seasoned seafood to the pot and simmer another 5 to 10 minutes, until the fish is cooked through. Discard the bay leaf.

5. Ladle the soup into bowls and garnish each serving with a tablespoon of cheese and a sprinkling of parsley or cilantro.

Meat Week Variation: Omit the cheese.

Maintenance Variation: Serve with 2 slices (about 1-inch thick) crusty French baguette.

FISH AND PEPPERS PACKETS

Serves 4

This recipe originally appeared in our book *The Low Carb CookwoRx Cookbook* (Wiley, 2005).

1 to 2 tablespoons extra-virgin olive oil

4 pieces (4 to 5 ounces each) salmon, sea bass, or other firm fish

1 teaspoon salt, or more to taste

1 teaspoon black pepper, or more to taste

½ teaspoon ground cumin

½ yellow bell pepper, seeded and coarsely diced

½ red bell pepper, seeded and coarsely diced

1 poblano or pasilla chile (or green bell pepper), seeded and sliced into 8 to 12 rings

2 medium zucchini, sliced lengthwise and diced

½ medium white onion, sliced

1 tablespoon minced fresh basil, or 1 teaspoon dried

2 tablespoons minced fresh cilantro, or 2 teaspoons dried

1. Preheat the oven to 425° F.

2. Tear 4 rectangles of aluminum foil large enough to make loose packets to hold the fish and vegetables. Lightly oil the central area of each piece of foil.

3. Rinse the fish and pat dry with a paper towel. Remove the skin; find any stray bones by running your finger tip along the flesh and remove them with a pair of tweezers.

4. Place a piece of fish in the center of each foil rectangle. Sprinkle each piece lightly with salt, pepper, and cumin.

5. Distribute the peppers, zucchini, and onion slices evenly over the fish pieces. Sprinkle with the herbs and drizzle with the remaining olive oil.

6. Fold the foil ends together and crimp the middle and both ends to make a sealed packet. Place the packets on a baking sheet and bake for 20 to 25 minutes. Serve immediately.

SEARED AHI TUNA

Serves 2

¼ *cup soy sauce*

1 *tablespoon grated fresh ginger*

¼ *teaspoon dry mustard*

½ *teaspoon wasabi powder*

¼ *cup sesame oil*

2 *(3- to 4-ounce) pieces sashimi-grade ahi tuna, about 2 inches thick*

2 *tablespoons white sesame seeds*

2 *tablespoons black sesame seeds*

2 *cups mixed salad lettuces*

1. In a bowl, combine the soy sauce, ginger, mustard, and wasabi. Stream in the sesame oil, whisking constantly, to make a light dressing. Set about 2 tablespoons of the dressing aside.

2. Place the tuna in a large zipper-sealed plastic bag and pour the remaining dressing over, turning to coat evenly. Seal and let the tuna marinate at least 20 minutes at room temperature or up to overnight in the refrigerator. (Also refrigerate the reserved dressing, sealed in a small container, if you marinate the fish overnight.)

3. Oil a cold grill pan, griddle, or charcoal or gas grill grate, and heat grill to very hot.

4. In a shallow bowl or pie plate, mix the black and white sesame seeds.

5. Drain marinade from tuna, but leave it wet. Lay each piece of tuna in the sesame seeds and press lightly; flip and repeat to coat both sides.

6. Place the tuna on the hot grill and sear each side, 1 to 2 minutes, for a rare to medium-rare interior.

7. Dress the salad greens lightly with the reserved dressing, then lay the seared ahi on top and serve.

GRILLED CITRUS-ROSEMARY SALMON

Serves 2

1 tablespoon white wine vinegar

Juice and zest from 1 lime

1 teaspoon chopped fresh rosemary (or ½ teaspoon dried)

1 teaspoon chopped fresh parsley (or ½ teaspoon dried)

¼ teaspoon garlic powder

½ teaspoon sea salt

¼ teaspoon freshly ground black pepper

3 tablespoons olive oil

2 (6- to 8-ounce) salmon fillets or steaks

1. In a small bowl, whisk together the vinegar, lime juice, zest, rosemary, parsley, garlic powder, salt, and pepper. Let sit for 15 minutes for flavors to combine.

2. Meanwhile, rinse the fillets and pat dry. Remove any small bones. Place the fillets into a zipper-sealed plastic bag.

3. Whisk the olive oil into the citrus-and-spice mixture to make a marinade and pour all but 2 tablespoons of the mixture over the fish fillets. Reserve the small amount of marinade to dress the fish after cooking. Seal the bag and allow fish to marinate in the refrigerator for at least 1 hour and up to overnight.

4. Grill the fish over medium-high heat for 4 minutes per inch of thickness, skin side down. Flip and cook another 3 to 4 minutes.

5. Remove to a serving plate and drizzle with the reserved citrus marinade.

SHRIMP SALAD–STUFFED AVOCADO

Serves 2

Juice of 1 lime
¼ teaspoon salt
¼ teaspoon freshly ground black pepper
1 teaspoon ketchup
2 tablespoons Basic Blender Mayonnaise (page 272)
1 can (5 ounces) tiny shrimp, drained
1 celery stalk, finely diced
¼ medium sweet onion (Vidalia, Maui, or the like), finely diced
1 Hass avocado (the largest ripe one available)
2 large lettuce leaves (red leaf, Bibb, or other)
Salt and pepper
Extra-virgin olive oil

1. In a bowl, combine half the lime juice with the salt, pepper, ketchup, and mayonnaise and stir to blend well.

2. Add the shrimp, celery, and onion and toss to coat.

3. Cut the avocado in half lengthwise, remove the seed, and using a large serving spoon, carefully scoop the pulp out of each half, keeping the half intact.

4. Discard the shells. Sprinkle the remaining lime juice over the avocado and gently rub the halves to spread the juice across the surface.

5. Place each avocado half on a lettuce leaf, sprinkle lightly with salt and pepper, and drizzle with a bit of olive oil.

6. Mound half the shrimp salad onto each avocado half and serve.

Flavor Variations: Substitute a drained can of tuna or ¾ cup diced cooked chicken for the shrimp.

Maintenance Variation: Slice the avocado half and place it, the shrimp salad, and the lettuce leaf in a warmed flour tortilla.

SPEEDY GARLIC SHRIMP

Serves 4 to 6

1 cup (2 sticks) butter
¼ cup plus 1 teaspoon Worcestershire sauce
½ teaspoon garlic powder
½ teaspoon black pepper
Few dashes of Tabasco or other hot pepper sauce
3 pounds shrimp deveined with tails on, rinsed and dried
Pinch of salt

1. Place the butter, Worcestershire sauce, garlic powder, pepper, and Tabasco sauce in a microwave-safe bowl, cover with a paper towel, and microwave on high for 1 to 2 minutes, or until butter is melted.

2. Place the shrimp in a large microwave-safe bowl or casserole dish, pour the melted butter over them, and toss to coat. Cover the bowl with a paper towel and microwave on 80 percent power for 10 to 12 minutes, or until opaque.

3. Taste shrimp for seasoning upon removal. If needed, sprinkle on a pinch of salt, toss lightly, and serve.

VEGETABLES AND FRUITS

BROCCOLI AMONDINE

Serves 4

1 tablespoon butter

1 tablespoon olive oil

1 garlic clove, crushed, but whole

2 cups broccoli florets, washed and drained

¼ cup vegetable broth or water

¼ cup slivered blanched almonds

½ teaspoon salt, or to taste

¼ teaspoon ground black pepper

1. In a skillet, heat the butter and oil over medium heat until melted and add the garlic; sauté 2 or 3 minutes.

2. Add the broccoli, stir to coat with the oil, and sauté for 2 minutes.

3. Add the broth, cover the skillet, and cook another 4 minutes.

4. Remove the cover, stir in the almonds, salt, and pepper, and cook only until the liquid has evaporated, about 2 to 3 minutes more.

5. Serve immediately.

PARMESAN BROCCOLI AND RED PEPPERS

Serves 4

2 cups broccoli florets, washed and well drained

1 tablespoon olive oil

1 tablespoon butter

1 garlic clove, finely minced

½ teaspoon salt

¼ teaspoon black pepper

½ cup vegetable broth

2 canned roasted red peppers, rinsed, seeded, and cut into lengthwise strips

¼ cup freshly grated Parmesan cheese

1. Cut the broccoli florets in half and also slice any very large florets lengthwise again.

2. Heat the olive oil and butter in a large skillet over medium heat. Add the garlic and sauté for 1 minute to infuse the oil with flavor.

3. Add the broccoli, salt, and pepper and stir to coat with the oil. Sauté for 2 minutes.

4. Add the broth, cover the skillet, and steam the broccoli until tender, about 4 minutes.

5. Remove the cover, stir in the red peppers, and continue cooking until all liquid is gone, about another 2 to 3 minutes.

6. Sprinkle on the cheese, toss, and serve.

Meat Week Variation: Omit the cheese from the recipe.

BROILED HERBED TOMATO HALVES

Serves 4

4 Roma or plum tomatoes
1 tablespoon olive oil, plus additional for baking dish
Sea salt and freshly ground black pepper to taste
1 teaspoon finely chopped fresh rosemary, or ½ teaspoon dried
1 teaspoon finely chopped fresh parsley, or ½ teaspoon dried
1 garlic clove, finely minced

1. Preheat the broiler to high.

2. Cut each tomato in half lengthwise. Drizzle the cut surfaces with olive oil and lightly salt and pepper them.

3. Mix the herbs and garlic and divide evenly among the 8 halves, spreading the mixture across their surfaces.

4. Place the halves in a lightly oiled baking dish and broil for 5 or 6 minutes, or until tomatoes begin to soften and brown slightly.

Maintenance Variation: Sprinkle grated Parmigiano-Reggiano cheese over the tomatoes before broiling.

HONEY MUSTARD GREEN BEANS

Serves 4

1 (16-ounce) bag frozen whole green beans, thawed

1 tablespoon olive oil

½ teaspoon sea salt

¼ teaspoon freshly ground black pepper

1 tablespoon Dijon mustard

2 teaspoons soy sauce

1 packet Splenda or stevia

1. Preheat the oven to 450° F.

2. Drain the green beans of any excess water and pat dry with a paper towel.

3. Drizzle the beans with olive oil, sprinkle on salt and pepper, and toss to coat.

4. Spread the beans in a single layer on a foil-lined baking sheet, and bake for 15 to 20 minutes, stirring every 5 minutes, until tender and slightly browned.

5. In a small bowl, whisk together the mustard, soy sauce, and sweetener.

6. When the beans are cooked, drizzle on the mustard mixture, toss to coat, and return to the oven for another 4 or 5 minutes.

7. Serve hot.

CREAMY CAULIFLOWER PUREE

Serves 4

1 large head cauliflower

2 tablespoons butter, melted

½ Boursin Cheese with Herbs and Garlic, at room temperature

1 to 2 tablespoons heavy cream

½ teaspoon salt, or to taste

¼ teaspoon pepper, or to taste

1. Wash the cauliflower and trim away tough outer leaves. Slice the head in half once and then again to make 4 pieces. Cut each piece into ½-inch slices.

2. Place the cauliflower in a microwave-safe bowl, cover, and microwave on high for 6 minutes. Stir and microwave on high for another 3 minutes. Allow cauliflower to cool slightly.

3. Place the cooked cauliflower into the workbowl of a food processor. Add the melted butter, cheese, 1 tablespoon of the cream, and the salt and pepper. Process in pulses to start and then on high until smooth. Add more cream if needed to achieve a smooth puree that holds its shape like mashed potatoes.

4. Adjust seasonings if needed, and serve. (Will keep warm, covered, for up to 30 minutes in the microwave on "keep warm" if your oven has that setting or over a pan of simmering water.)

FRIED CAULI-RICE

Serves 4

1 head cauliflower, washed and trimmed of leaves

2 large eggs

2 tablespoons organic lard, bacon fat, or sesame oil

2 green onions, white and green parts, chopped

1 garlic clove, minced

¼ teaspoon red chile paste (see Note)

¼ cup frozen green peas

1 roasted red pepper (jarred or canned), finely chopped

2 tablespoons soy sauce

1. Cut the cauliflower into chunks and put into the workbowl of a food processor fitted with a steel blade. Process in pulses until you've got "rice size" pieces.

2. Place the chopped cauliflower into a microwave-safe bowl, cover, and microwave on high for 4 to 5 minutes, until tender-crisp. (Use only the water still clinging to the cauliflower; don't add any.)

3. Beat the eggs lightly.

4. Heat the fat in a large skillet or wok until nearly smoking. Pour the eggs into the pan and stir constantly until they are scrambled, but not dry. Remove from the pan to a paper towel–lined bowl.

5. Drop the green onions, garlic, and chile paste into the pan and stir-fry for about 1 minute, then add the cauliflower, peas, pepper, and soy sauce. Heat through, about another minute or two.

6. Return the scrambled eggs to the pan and stir to thoroughly combine, then serve.

Note: Red chile paste is available in the international foods aisle of most grocery stores. If you can't find it, substitute ⅛ teaspoon Tabasco sauce or cayenne pepper or ½ teaspoon red pepper flakes.

HERBED CAULI-RICE

Serves 4

1 head cauliflower, washed and trimmed of leaves

2 tablespoons olive oil or melted butter

1 garlic clove, finely minced

1 tablespoon minced fresh mint

1 tablespoon minced fresh basil

1 tablespoon minced fresh flat-leaf parsley

¼ teaspoon coarse sea salt

¼ teaspoon black pepper

1. Cut the cauliflower into chunks and put into the workbowl of a food processor fitted with a steel blade. Process in pulses until you've got "rice size" pieces.

2. Place the chopped cauliflower into a microwave-safe bowl, cover, and microwave on high for 5 to 6 minutes, until tender. (Use only the water clinging to the vegetable; don't add any.)

3. Heat the oil in a large skillet over medium heat. Add the garlic and sauté briefly, just to soften. Do not brown.

4. Add the cauliflower, herbs, salt, and pepper and stir to combine well. Cook until heated through, about 2 minutes.

5. Serve immediately. (Store leftovers in a tightly covered container for up to a week.)

Time-saving Tip: Make a double batch; store in refrigerator for use in soups, salads, or side dishes for up to a week.

CRUNCHY CABBAGE SLAW

Serves 4 to 6

¾ cup distilled white vinegar

½ teaspoon salt

¼ teaspoon black pepper

½ teaspoon celery seeds

½ teaspoon dry mustard

4 packets Splenda

2 cups packaged cabbage slaw mix (green cabbage, red cabbage, carrots)

½ green bell pepper, seeded and diced

½ small red onion, diced

1. In a large bowl, whisk together the vinegar, salt, pepper, celery seeds, mustard, and Splenda.

2. Add the slaw mix, bell pepper, and red onion and toss to coat evenly.

3. Cover and refrigerate at least 1 hour or overnight.

Time-saving Tip: Make a double batch; it will keep in the refrigerator for several days, covered.

Flavor Variation: Substitute broccoli slaw for the cabbage slaw for an equally delicious but different taste.

SAUTÉED APPLES AND RED CABBAGE

Serves 4

1½ teaspoons kosher salt (not sea salt)
1 small red cabbage, cored and tough outer leaves removed, chopped
1 tart apple (Granny Smith or similar), peeled, cored, and diced
Juice of 1 lemon
1 tablespoon olive oil
1 tablespoon butter
¼ medium white onion, diced
¼ teaspoon garlic powder
½ teaspoon dry mustard
¼ teaspoon black pepper
2 packets Splenda or other noncaloric, heat-stable sweetener

1. Bring a large pot of water to a rolling boil, add 1 teaspoon salt, and gently drop the cabbage into the pot. Cook for 2 minutes, remove from the heat, and drain.

2. Place the apple dice in a bowl and douse with lemon juice; toss to coat.

3. In a large skillet, heat the olive oil and butter over medium heat. Add the onion, apple, seasonings, and Splenda, and sauté, stirring to prevent scorching, until softened slightly, about 3 minutes.

4. Add the cabbage, toss to combine while heating through, then serve.

Time-saving Tip: Double the batch if your skillet permits. This recipe keeps well in the refrigerator and reheats easily in the microwave.

SAVORY SAUTÉED APPLE SLICES

Serves 2

1 medium apple (Gala, Fuji, Granny Smith, or other)
Juice and zest of 1 lemon
¼ teaspoon ground cinnamon
⅛ teaspoon ground allspice
Dash of sea salt
1 packet Splenda, stevia, or other noncaloric, heat-stable sweetener
2 tablespoons butter
Whipped cream (unsweetened or artificially sweetened; optional)

1. Peel, core, and slice the apple. Place the slices in a bowl and douse with the lemon juice, stirring to coat.

2. Add the spices, salt, and sweetener and stir to coat slices evenly.

3. Melt the butter in a small skillet over medium-high heat. When it foams, add the apple slices and sauté, stirring frequently, until softened, about 3 to 4 minutes.

4. Serve warm with a dollop of whipped cream, if desired.

Time-saving Tip: Make a double, triple, or even quadruple batch. Refrigerate the extra servings in small snap-lid, microwave-safe containers for up to a week. (To reheat, microwave about 2 minutes on 50 percent power and 30-second bursts on high, stirring between, until heated through.)

GRILLED PLUMS, NECTARINES, OR PEACHES

Serves 4

Instead of making the reduction, you can substitute a drizzle of Villa Mandori Aceto Balsamico straight from the bottle, since it's already very thick and delicious, if a little pricey.

3 tablespoons balsamic vinegar

1 packet Splenda or stevia

3 or 4 grinds of fresh black pepper, plus more for serving

2 large ripe plums, nectarines, or peaches, washed and patted dry

1 teaspoon olive oil

1. Preheat a charcoal or gas grill or a grill pan on the stovetop.

2. Place the balsamic vinegar, sweetener, and black pepper into a small saucepan over medium heat and reduce by half or a little more, to about 1 tablespoon.

3. Wash the fruit and pat dry. Split in half and remove the pits.

4. Lightly brush each cut surface with olive oil and grill for 5 to 7 minutes over medium-high heat. Place cut side up on a plate, and drizzle with the balsamic reduction. Grind a bit of black pepper over the fruit just before serving.

CHILLED FRUIT SOUP

Serves 6

½ cup Sweet Orange Water (recipe follows)

2 cups seeded cubed watermelon

1 package (10 ounces) frozen raspberries, thawed

½ cup plain yogurt

Juice of 1 lime

1 teaspoon minced fresh ginger

1 cup peeled and diced ripe cantaloupe

1 bunch fresh mint, for garnish

1. In a blender (working in batches, if necessary) puree all the ingredients except the cantaloupe until smooth and thick. (Add a bit of extra water, if needed, to achieve a thinner consistency, if desired.)

2. Refrigerate the soup for at least 30 minutes or up to several hours.

3. To serve, ladle soup into bowls, top with pieces of diced cantaloupe, and garnish with a sprig of fresh mint.

SWEET ORANGE WATER

½ cup water

Zest of 1 orange, grated

8 packets Splenda, stevia, or equivalent noncaloric sweetener

1. Place the water in a small saucepan; add the orange zest and the sweetener and bring to a boil.

2. Turn off the heat and let the mixture infuse for 30 minutes at room temperature, or place the mixture in a container with a tight-fitting lid and infuse overnight in the refrigerator.

STRAWBERRY, MANDARIN, AND MINT CUP

Serves 4 to 6

2 cups stemmed and sliced fresh strawberries

1 can (4 ounces) mandarin orange segments, drained

Juice and zest of 1 lime

1 tablespoon chopped fresh mint leaves

1 packet Splenda, stevia, or other noncaloric sweetener

1. Combine all the ingredients in a bowl and toss well.
2. Cover and chill for at least 30 minutes before serving.

MIXED FRUIT SALAD

Serves 6

1 cup fresh raspberries
1 cup diced cantaloupe
1 cup diced honeydew
½ cup fresh blackberries
1 kiwi, peeled and diced
4 ounces plain yogurt
3 packets Splenda or stevia
Juice and zest of 1 lime
½ teaspoon poppy seeds

1. Combine all the fruit in a large serving bowl.

2. In a small bowl, whisk together the yogurt, sweetener, lime juice and zest, and poppy seeds.

3. Just at serving time, pour the dressing over the fruit and toss to coat evenly.

JUST A FEW SWEET TREATS

There aren't many sweet treats in this recipe collection, primarily because during the six weeks of The Cure we have chiefly used fresh fruits, such as berries and melons, as the preferred choices in our meal plans. Also, we encourage you to use this time to curb your sweet tooth. While you might want or need a sweet treat now and again, we recommend, by and large, that you put off eating sweets until the maintenance stage, because the surest way to undermine your fat-loss and weight-loss efforts is to fill up on low-carb or no-carb calories. While the recipes here don't have much in the way of sugar or carbohydrate, they're quite calorie rich and ought, like all sweets, to be used infrequently and in moderation.

You can find many more recipes for sweets (and a ton of other dishes) in our two cookbooks, *The Low Carb Comfort Cookbook* (Wiley, 2003), which we coauthored with Ursula Solom, and in the companion book to our PBS television cooking show, *The Low Carb CookwoRx Cookbook* (Wiley, 2005).

HOMEMADE VANILLA ICE CREAM

Makes about 1 quart (16 servings)

2 large eggs, pasteurized in the shell
⅔ cup granular Splenda or its equivalent
2 cups heavy cream
1½ cups half-and-half
¼ cup nonfat dry milk powder
2 teaspoons vanilla extract

1. In a large bowl, beat the eggs and Splenda until pale yellow.

2. Add the cream, half-and-half, dry milk, and vanilla and beat until thoroughly mixed.

3. Pour the mixture into an ice cream maker and process according to the manufacturer's directions.

4. Place the ice cream in a freezer-safe container and store in your freezer at least 30 minutes to 1 hour to firm the consistency before serving.

Flavor Variations: For strawberry ice cream, roughly puree 1 cup (thawed) frozen unsweetened strawberries, leaving some chunks. Substitute the puree for 1 cup of the half-and-half. Increase the amount of Splenda by 2 tablespoons. For dulce de leche ice cream, substitute ½ cup Torini or DaVinci Sugar-Free Caramel Syrup for ½ cup of the half-and-half and reduce the Splenda to ½ cup.

GUILT-FREE MINI-CHEESECAKES

Serves 6

8 ounces cream cheese (organic, if possible)
½ cup sour cream (organic, if possible)
½ cup half-and-half (organic, if possible)
2 large eggs
3 packets Splenda, stevia, or other noncaloric sweetener
2 teaspoons vanilla extract

FOR THE CRUST

6 tablespoons finely chopped walnuts, pecans, or hazelnuts
2 packets Splenda, stevia, or other noncaloric sweetener of your choice
1 tablespoon butter, melted

1. Preheat the oven to 350° F. Lightly grease the cups of a 6-cup muffin tin with butter.

2. In a blender or food processor, combine the cream cheese, sour cream, half-and-half, eggs, sweetener, and vanilla and blend until smooth.

3. In a small bowl, combine the chopped nuts, sweetener, and melted butter.

4. Place 1 tablespoon of the nut mixture into each muffin cup and press into an even layer. Fill each cup about three-fourth full with the cream cheese mixture.

5. Bake for 25 minutes or until a toothpick inserted in the center comes out clean. Remove, cool slightly, then cover with plastic wrap or waxed paper and chill in the refrigerator for at least several hours. (These will keep, sealed in a snap-lid container, for several days in the refrigerator.)

Flavor Variations

- Berry Cheesecakes. Top baked cheesecakes with ¼ cup thawed unsweetened berries, mashed slightly, with an additional packet of sweetener and a tablespoon of lemon or lime juice.
- Chocolate chip cheesecakes. Substitute ¼ cup mini-chocolate chips for half the sour cream.
- Lemon cheesecakes. Substitute 1 teaspoon lemon extract for 1 teaspoon of the vanilla and add 1 tablespoon lemon zest. At serving time, top with a very thin slice of lemon, a curl of lemon peel, and a dollop of Sweet Lime Cream (recipe follows) prepared with lemon.
- Caramel cheesecakes. Substitute ¼ cup of Torini or DaVinci Sugar-Free Caramel Syrup for half of the sour cream.
- Mocha cheesecakes. Add 1 tablespoon espresso powder to the cream cheese mixture and substitute ¼ cup mini–chocolate chips for half the sour cream.

SWEET LIME CREAM

Serves 4 to 6

½ cup heavy whipping cream (organic, if possible)
Zest of 1 lime
2 packets Splenda, stevia, or other noncaloric sweetener

In a chilled bowl, whip the cream until soft peaks form. Add the sweetener and zest, and continue to whip until slight firmer. Use immediately if possible. (But this will keep, covered, in the refrigerator for up to 30 minutes.)

Flavor Variation: Replace the lime zest with orange or lemon zest, or replace the zest with ½ teaspoon vanilla, almond, banana, coconut, or maple extract.

SAUCES, CONDIMENTS, AND DRESSINGS

BASIC BLENDER MAYONNAISE

Makes about 1 cup

For safety, in recipes calling for raw eggs, use eggs pasteurized in their shells. Many grocery stores carry them, or your grocer can order them for you. If they're not available, prior to their use, immerse the egg in its shell in boiling water for 30 seconds.

1 large egg yolk, pasteurized in the shell
1 teaspoon dry mustard
1 teaspoon sea salt
Dash of cayenne pepper
1 packet Splenda, stevia, or other noncaloric sweetener (optional)
1 tablespoon lemon juice or champagne vinegar
¾ to 1 cup light olive oil

1. In a blender jar, combine the egg yolk, mustard, salt, cayenne, and sweetener on high speed for 30 seconds. Add the lemon juice and blend again.

2. In a slow, steady stream, with the motor running, add the olive oil until the emulsion will hold no more oil and the mayonnaise is firm enough to stand on its own.

3. Store in the refrigerator in a container with a tight-fitting lid for up to a week.

CAESAR DRESSING

Serves 4

Juice of 1 lemon

1 garlic clove

4 anchovy fillets (boneless, if possible), or 1½ teaspoons anchovy paste

1 tablespoon Basic Blender Mayonnaise (page 272)

1 tablespoon Dijon mustard

1 tablespoon Worcestershire sauce

1. Put the lemon juice into a shallow bowl.

2. Finely mince or press the garlic and add to the lemon juice.

3. Add the 4 anchovy fillets and mash with 2 forks until you've got a smooth paste (or use anchovy paste equal to 4 anchovies—1 to 1½ teaspoons).

4. Add the mayonnaise, mustard, and Worcestershire sauce and mix with a fork to blend thoroughly.

CREAMY GORGONZOLA DRESSING

Serves 8

¼ cup white wine vinegar

1 tablespoon chopped shallot

¼ teaspoon Dijon mustard

¼ teaspoon garlic powder

⅛ teaspoon Herbes de Provence

⅛ teaspoon freshly ground black pepper

½ cup heavy cream

2 ounces gorgonzola cheese, crumbled (¼ cup)

1. In a bowl, combine the vinegar, shallot, mustard, garlic powder, Herbes de Provence, and pepper. Let sit for 10 to 15 minutes to allow the flavors to infuse the vinegar.

2. Whisk in the cream in a slow stream. Add the cheese and stir to combine. Use immediately or store in a tightly sealed container in the refrigerator for up to 5 days.

MINTED YOGURT DRESSING

Serves 4

¼ *cup white wine vinegar*

2 *tablespoons finely chopped fresh mint*

1 *tablespoon finely chopped fresh flat-leaf parsley, or 1 teaspoon dried*

1 *tablespoon finely chopped fresh chives, or ½ teaspoon onion powder*

1 *garlic clove, finely minced*

¼ *teaspoon salt, or to taste*

¼ *teaspoon black pepper, or to taste*

½ *cup plain yogurt*

¼ *cup heavy cream*

1. Combine the vinegar, herbs, garlic, salt, and pepper in a bowl and allow the mixture to sit for 15 minutes or longer to meld the flavors.

2. Mix in the yogurt and cream, whisking to blend thoroughly. You can use immediately, but if possible place in a container with a tight-fitting lid and refrigerate for 1 hour to further develop the flavor. The dressing will keep, refrigerated, for up to 1 week.

DIJON VINAIGRETTE

Serves 4

Juice and zest of ½ lemon
1 tablespoon champagne vinegar
1 teaspoon Dijon mustard
½ teaspoon sea salt
¼ teaspoon freshly ground black pepper
⅓ cup extra-virgin olive oil

1. In a bowl, combine all the ingredients except the oil and allow to sit for a few minutes.

2. Whisk in the oil in a slow steady stream. Use immediately or store in a snap-lid container or jar with a tight-fitting lid in the refrigerator for several days. Bring to room temperature before serving; whisk or shake vigorously to reblend the oil if needed.

Time-saving Tip: Make a double batch of vinaigrette and store in the refrigerator for use all week.

MINTED VINEGAR

Makes ½ cup

4 ounces malt vinegar

4 packets Splenda or stevia

2 tablespoons finely chopped fresh mint

1. In a small saucepan, combine the vinegar and sweetener and bring to a boil over medium-high heat.

2. Remove from heat, stir in the mint, and allow the mixture to cool to room temperature.

3. Pour the minted vinegar into a sealed container and refrigerate for at least an hour. The vinegar will keep, refrigerated, for several days.

LOW-CARB BÉCHAMEL SAUCE

Makes about 1 cup

1 tablespoon unsalted butter

1 teaspoon ThickenThin not/Starch

1 cup heavy cream

¼ teaspoon sea salt

⅛ teaspoon white pepper

Pinch of freshly grated nutmeg

1. In a saucepan, melt the butter over medium-high heat. Make a roux by adding the ThickenThin and whisking until smooth, 30 seconds to 1 minute. Do not let the roux brown.

2. Slowly whisk in the cream until the sauce becomes smooth and thick, 2 or 3 minutes, but do not let it boil.

3. Season with salt, pepper, and nutmeg, reduce the heat, and simmer for a couple of minutes before using.

Flavor Variation: For Low-Carb Mornay Sauce, add ¼ cup grated cheese (Gruyère, Parmesan, white Cheddar, Emmenthaler, fontina) and stir until melted. Thin (if needed) with just a little milk and serve immediately atop steamed fresh veggies or seafood.

CRANBERRY-ORANGE RELISH

Makes about 24 heaping tablespoons

This recipe has been adapted with permission from *Low Carb CookwoRx Cookbook* (Wiley, 2005).

1 large orange

1½ cups fresh cranberries (about ½ package)

¾ cup granulated Splenda

1. Wash and trim the stem ends from the orange and quarter it.

2. Zest the orange, then peel or cut away the white pith and cut the flesh into quarters. Place the orange, zest, cranberries, and Splenda into the workbowl of a food processor fitted with a steel blade.

3. Pulse to chop the orange and berries to a fine mince.

4. Taste for sweetness. Depending on the sweetness of the fruit, you may wish to add another 1 to 2 tablespoons of Splenda, although it should be tangy. (Remember that each tablespoon of additional granulated Splenda will add 3 grams of carbohydrate to the recipe total.)

5. Turn the mixture into a pretty serving bowl, cover tightly with plastic wrap, and refrigerate overnight if possible to develop more intense flavor.

6. Serve cold. The relish will keep, tightly covered, in the refrigerator for up to a week.

APPENDIX

TABLE I **FOOD SUBSTITUTIONS LIST, VEGETABLES**

Artichoke, boiled—½

Artichoke hearts, marinated—
    ½ cup

Asparagus—6–8 spears

Bamboo shoots—1 cup

Beans, green, canned or frozen—
    ½ cup

Beans, wax, canned—½ cup

Beets—½ cup

Black soy beans—½ cup

Broccoli—2 cups

Brussels sprouts—7 or 8

Carrot, raw—1 medium

Carrot, cooked—½ cup

Cauliflower, raw—1 cup

Cauliflower, cooked, puree—½ cup

Coleslaw—½ cup (no-sugar)

Eggplant, cooked—½ cup

Greens, boiled—1 cup (mustard,
    turnip, collard, kale, chard)

Leeks, boiled—½ cup

Mushrooms, raw—2 cups

Mushrooms, cooked—1 cup

Okra, boiled—1 cup

Onion, yellow, raw chopped—
    ½ cup

Onions, green, raw—½ cup

Peas, green—½ cup, canned

Peppers, chile—1 whole (pasilla,
    poblano)

Peppers, sweet bell—½ large

Pumpkin, cooked—½ cup

Rhubarb, cooked—1 cup

Rutabaga, boiled—½ cup

Sauerkraut, canned—½ cup

Shallots, chopped—3 tablespoons

Squash, summer, cooked—½ cup

Squash, winter, cooked—½ cup

Tomatillo—3 whole

Tomato, medium, raw—1

Tomato, canned—½ cup

Tomato, sun-dried—¼ cup

Turnips, boiled—½ cup

TABLE 2 **FOOD SUBSTITUTIONS LIST, FRUITS**

Apple, raw—½

Apple, cooked—⅓ cup

Applesauce—⅓ cup

Apricot, canned—4 halves

Avocado, Hass—1 medium

Blackberries—¾ cup

Blueberries—½ cup

Cantaloupe—¾ cup

Cherries, sour, canned (in water)—
   ¼ cup

Cranberries, raw—½ cup

Currants, black, raw—½ cup

Currants, black, dried—
   1 tablespoon

Dates—1

Figs, raw—½ medium

Fruit cocktail, canned (in water)—
   ¼ cup

Grapefruit, raw—½

Grapefruit, canned—⅓ cup

Grapes—½ cup

Guava, raw—½ medium

Honeydew melon—½ cup

Kiwifruit—1 medium

Nectarine—½ medium

Orange, mandarin, raw—1 small

Orange, mandarin, canned—⅓ cup

Orange, Valencia or navel—
   ½ small

Papaya, raw—¼ medium

Passionfruit, raw—1 medium

Peach, raw—½ medium

Peach, canned (in water)—⅓ cup

Pear, raw—½ medium

Pear, canned (in water)—⅓ cup

Persimmon, raw—1 medium

Pineapple, raw—½ cup

Pineapple, canned (in water)—
   ¼ cup

Plum, raw—1 medium

Raspberries, fresh—1 cup

Strawberries, fresh—1 cup

Watermelon—¾ cup

TABLE 3 **MEAT WEEKS FOOD SUBSTITUTIONS LIST, VEGETABLES**

Artichoke, boiled—½

Artichoke hearts, marinated—
   ½ cup

Asparagus—6–8 spears

Bamboo shoots—1 cup

Beans, green, canned or frozen—
   ½ cup

Beans, wax, canned—½ cup

Broccoli—2 cups

Brussels sprouts—7 or 8

Cauliflower, raw—1 cup

Cauliflower, cooked, puree—½ cup

Coleslaw—½ cup (no-sugar)

Greens, boiled—1 cup (mustard,
   turnip, collard, kale, chard)

Leeks, boiled—½ cup

Mushrooms, raw—1 cup

Mushrooms, cooked—1 cup

Okra, boiled—½ cup

Onions, green, raw—¼ cup

Peppers, chile—1 (pasilla, poblano)

Peppers, sweet bell—½ large

Rhubarb, cooked—¼ cup

Sauerkraut, canned—½ cup

Shallots, chopped—3 tablespoons

Squash, summer—½ cup

Tomatillo—3 whole

Tomato, raw, medium—1

Tomato, canned—½ cup

Tomato, sun-dried—¼ cup

TABLE 4 MEAT WEEKS FOOD SUBSTITUTIONS LIST, FRUITS

Avocado, Hass—1 medium

Blackberries—⅓ cup

Blueberries—¼ cup

Cantaloupe—⅛ small (1 slice)

Grapefruit, canned—¼ cup

Grapes—⅓ cup

Honeydew melon—⅛ small (1 slice)

Kiwifruit—½ medium

Nectarine—½ small

Orange, Valencia—½ small

Peach, raw—½ small

Pineapple, raw—¼ cup

Pineapple, canned (in water)— ⅛ cup

Plum, raw—½ small

Raspberries, fresh—½ cup

Strawberries, fresh—½ cup

TABLE 5 LEUCINE CONTENT OF FOODS

Food	Leucine Content (grams/3 ounces)
Soybeans (mature seeds, raw)	2.97
Beef (round, top round, raw)	1.76
Beef (top sirloin, raw)	1.74
Peanuts (all types)	1.67
Salami (Italian, pork)	1.63
Salmon (pink, raw)	1.62
Shrimp (mixed species, raw)	1.61
Chicken (dark meat, raw)	1.48
Almonds	1.47
Egg yolk (fresh, raw)	1.4
Sesame butter (tahini)	1.36
Chicken (white meat, raw)	1.29
Egg, whole (raw)	1.09
Egg, white (raw)	0.96

INITIAL ASSESSMENT AND PROGRESS LOG

Date			
Height			
Weight			
Waist			
Hips			
S-SAD			
L-SAD			
S-SAD minus L-SAD			
Body Fat %			
BP			
Blood Tests			
Fasting glulcose			
Hemoglobin A1c			
Fasting Insulin			
Total Cholesterol			
HDL Cholesterol			
LDL Cholesterol			
Triglycerides			
APO-B			
Lipoprotein (a)			
hs-TSH			
Iodine Saturation			
Ferritin			
hs-C-Reactive Protein			
Liver enzymes			
Salivary Cortisol			
Sex hormones			
Estrogens E1,2,3			
Progesterone			
Testosterone			
Other Tests:			

TABLE 6 INTERPRETING YOUR SAD MEASUREMENTS

Standing Sagittal Abdominal Diameter and Risk for Cardiovascular Disease

	Lowest Risk			Highest Risk
Women	<6.5 inches	7.4 inches	8.4 inches	>10 inches
Men	<7 inches	8.3 inches	9 inches	>10.6 inches

* From *American Journal of Epidemiology* (2006), 164(12), pp. 1,150–1,159

RESOURCES

- Calculate the caloric expenditure of various tasks:
  www.exrx.net/Calculators/Calories.html
- Sleep hygeine quiz (how well do you sleep?):
  www.ualr.edu/psycinfo/sleeph.htm
- Abdominal caliper use: www.6weekcure.com
- Blender bottle for making shakes: www.6weekcure.com
- Best shake blender on the market: www.blendtec.com (like having
  a Starbucks frapuccino machine in your kitchen)

PRODUCTS

- Natural remedies for acid reflux: www.protexid.com,
  www.6weekcure.com

- Flavorings and extracts by the dozen: www.spicebarn.com
- Leucine powder: www.6weekcure.com; www.cheapvitamins.com
- PowerUp! Shake powder: www.6weekcure.com
- Sugar Free Original Oregon Chai: www.worldpantry.com

LAB TESTS AND HORMONES

We have no affiliation with the following organizations, but have met with them or used their services ourselves and trust their expertise in this area.

- Guidance in bio-identical hormonal therapies and compounding pharmacy: www.signaturepharmacy.com www.sanysidropharmacy.com
- Referral to a bio-identical hormone compounding pharmacy near you: The International Academy of Compounding Pharmacists (IACP), www.iacpinfo@iacprx.org or call 1-800-927-4227.
- Hormone testing (saliva and blood spot): www.zrtlab.com
- Iodine Load Test: FFP Lab, 500 S. Allen Rd., Suite #1, Flat Rock, NC 28731; toll-free number, 1-877-900-5556
- Iodoral (oral iodine supplement): Optimox Research Corporation, 2720 Monterey Street, Suite 406, Torrance, CA 90503; toll-free number, 1-800-223-1601

BLOGS

- Our blogs and archives: www.proteinpower.com

BIBLIOGRAPHY

Adams, L. A., and P. Angulo. "Recent Concepts in Non-Alcoholic Fatty Liver Disease." *Diabet Med* 22, no. 9 (2005): 1129–33.

Ahima, R. S. "Insulin Resistance: Cause or Consequence of Nonalcoholic Steatohepatitis?" *Gastroenterology* 132, no. 1 (2007): 444–46.

Andersson, C. X., B. Gustafson, A. Hammarstedt, S. Hedjazifar, and U. Smith. "Inflamed Adipose Tissue, Insulin Resistance and Vascular Injury." *Diabetes Metab Res Rev* 24, no. 8 (2008): 595–603.

Andrews, R. D., D. A. MacLean, and S. E. Riechman. "Protein Intake for Skeletal Muscle Hypertrophy with Resistance Training in Seniors." *Int J Sport Nutr Exerc Metab* 16, no. 4 (2006): 362–72.

Andrews, R., P. Greenhaff, S. Curtis, A. Perry, and A. J. Cowley. "The Effect of Dietary Creatine Supplementation on Skeletal Muscle Metabolism in Congestive Heart Failure." *Eur Heart J* 19, no. 4 (1998): 617–22.

Barrett, Deirdre. *Waistland.* New York: W. W. Norton, 2007.

Benfield, L. L., K. R. Fox, D. M. Peters, H. Blake, I. Rogers, C. Grant, and A. Ness. "Magnetic Resonance Imaging of Abdominal Adiposity in a Large Cohort of British Children." *Int J Obes (Lond)* 32, no. 1 (2008): 91–99.

Benoit, S. C., D. J. Clegg, R. J. Seeley, and S. C. Woods. "Insulin and Leptin as Adiposity Signals." *Recent Prog Horm Res* 59 (2004): 267–85.

Bergman, R. N., S. P. Kim, K. J. Catalano, I. R. Hsu, J. D. Chiu, M. Kabir, K. Hucking, and M. Ader. "Why Visceral Fat Is Bad: Mechanisms of the Metabolic Syndrome." *Obesity (Silver Spring)* 14 Suppl 1 (2006): 16S–19S.

Bergman, R. N., S. P. Kim, I. R. Hsu, K. J. Catalano, J. D. Chiu, M. Kabir, J. M. Richey, and M. Ader. "Abdominal Obesity: Role in the Pathophysiology of Metabolic Disease and Cardiovascular Risk." *Am J Med* 120, no. 2 Suppl 1 (2007): S3–8; discussion S29–32.

Chaston, T. B., and J. B. Dixon. "Factors Associated with Percent Change in Visceral Versus Subcutaneous Abdominal Fat During Weight Loss: Findings from a Systematic Review." *Int J Obes (Lond)* 32, no. 4 (2008): 619–28.

Cheung, O., A. Kapoor, P. Puri, S. Sistrun, V. A. Luketic, C. C. Sargeant, M. J. Contos, M. L. Shiffman, R. T. Stravitz, R. K. Sterling, and A. J. Sanyal. "The Impact of Fat Distribution on the Severity of Nonalcoholic Fatty Liver Disease and Metabolic Syndrome." *Hepatology* 46, no. 4 (2007): 1091–100.

Clegg, D. J., L. M. Brown, S. C. Woods, and S. C. Benoit. "Gonadal Hormones Determine Sensitivity to Central Leptin and Insulin." *Diabetes* 55, no. 4 (2006): 978–87.

Coburn, J. W., D. J. Housh, T. J. Housh, M. H. Malek, T. W. Beck, J. T. Cramer, G. O. Johnson, and P. E. Donlin. "Effects of Leucine and Whey Protein Supplementation During Eight Weeks of Unilateral Resistance Training." *J Strength Cond Res* 20, no. 2 (2006): 284–91.

Day, C. P. "From Fat to Inflammation." *Gastroenterology* 130, no. 1 (2006): 207–10.

De Lorenzo, A., V. Del Gobbo, M. G. Premrov, M. Bigioni, F. Galvano, and L. Di Renzo. "Normal-Weight Obese Syndrome: Early Inflammation?" *Am J Clin Nutr* 85, no. 1 (2007): 40–45.

Di Renzo, L., V. Del Gobbo, M. Bigioni, M. G. Premrov, R. Cianci, and A. De Lorenzo. "Body Composition Analyses in Normal Weight Obese Women." *Eur Rev Med Pharmacol Sci* 10, no. 4 (2006): 191–96.

Donaldson, Blake F. *Strong Medicine*. Garden City: Doubleday, 1961.

Douds, A. C., and J. D. Maxwell. "Alcohol and the Heart: Good and Bad News." *Addiction* 89, no. 3 (1994): 259–61.

Eades, Michael R. *Thin So Fast*. New York: Warner Books, 1989.

Eades, Michael R., and Mary Dan Eades. *Protein Power*. New York: Bantam Books, 1996.

———. *The Protein Power Lifeplan*. New York: Warner Books, 2000.

Empana, J. P., P. Ducimetiere, M. A. Charles, and X. Jouven. "Sagittal Abdominal Diameter and Risk of Sudden Death in Asymptomatic Middle-Aged Men: The Paris Prospective Study I." *Circulation* 110, no. 18 (2004): 2781–85.

Epel, E. E., A. E. Moyer, C. D. Martin, S. Macary, N. Cummings, J. Rodin, and M. Rebuffe-Scrive. "Stress-Induced Cortisol, Mood, and Fat Distribution in Men." *Obes Res* 7, no. 1 (1999): 9–15.

Epel, E. S., B. McEwen, T. Seeman, K. Matthews, G. Castellazzo, K. D. Brownell, J. Bell, and J. R. Ickovics. "Stress and Body Shape: Stress-Induced Cortisol Secretion Is Consistently Greater among Women with Central Fat." *Psychosom Med* 62, no. 5 (2000): 623–32.

Evans, W. J. "Protein Nutrition, Exercise and Aging." *J Am Coll Nutr* 23, no. 6 Suppl (2004): 601S–609S.

Freedland, E. S. "Role of a Critical Visceral Adipose Tissue Threshold (Cvatt) in Metabolic Syndrome: Implications for Controlling Dietary Carbohydrates: A Review." *Nutr Metab (Lond)* 1, no. 1 (2004): 12.

Fruhbeck, G. "Does a Neat Difference in Energy Expenditure Lead to Obesity?" *Lancet* 366, no. 9486 (2005): 615–16.

Gazi, I. F., T. D. Filippatos, V. Tsimihodimos, V. G. Saougos, E. N. Liberopoulos, D. P. Mikhailidis, A. D. Tselepis, and M. Elisaf. "The Hypertriglyceridemic Waist Phenotype Is a Predictor of Elevated Levels of Small, Dense Ldl Cholesterol." *Lipids* 41, no. 7 (2006): 647–54.

Gentile, C. L., and M. J. Pagliassotti. "The Role of Fatty Acids in the Development and Progression of Nonalcoholic Fatty Liver Disease." *J Nutr Biochem* 19, no. 9 (2008): 567–76.

Ginsberg, H. N. "Is the Slippery Slope from Steatosis to Steatohepatitis Paved with Triglyceride or Cholesterol?" *Cell Metab* 4, no. 3 (2006): 179–81.

Gottschall, Jonathan. "Patterns of Characterization in Folktales across Geographica Regions and Levels of Cultural Complexity." *Human Nature* 14, no. 4 (2003): 365–82.

———. "The 'Beauty Myth' Is No Myth." *Human Nature* 19, no. 2 (2008): 174–88.

Gower, B. A., J. Munoz, R. Desmond, T. Hilario-Hailey, and X. Jiao. "Changes in Intra-Abdominal Fat in Early Postmenopausal Women: Effects of Hormone Use." *Obesity (Silver Spring)* 14, no. 6 (2006): 1046–55.

Gower, B. A., T. R. Nagy, M. I. Goran, M. J. Toth, and E. T. Poehlman. "Fat Distribution and Plasma Lipid-Lipoprotein Concentrations in Pre- and Postmenopausal Women." *Int J Obes Relat Metab Disord* 22, no. 7 (1998): 605–11.

Grammer, K., B. Fink, A. P. Moller, and R. Thornhill. "Darwinian Aesthetics: Sexual Selection and the Biology of Beauty." *Biol Rev Camb Philos Soc* 78, no. 3 (2003): 385–407.

Green, J. S., P. R. Stanforth, T. Rankinen, A. S. Leon, D. Rao Dc, J. S. Skinner, C. Bouchard, and J. H. Wilmore. "The Effects of Exercise Training on Abdominal

Visceral Fat, Body Composition, and Indicators of the Metabolic Syndrome in Post-menopausal Women with and without Estrogen Replacement Therapy: The Her-itage Family Study." *Metabolism* 53, no. 9 (2004): 1192–96.

Greenberg, J. A., C. C. Dunbar, R. Schnoll, R. Kokolis, S. Kokolis, and J. Kassotis. "Caf-feinated Beverage Intake and the Risk of Heart Disease Mortality in the Elderly: A Prospective Analysis." *Am J Clin Nutr* 85, no. 2 (2007): 392–98.

Gustafson, B., A. Hammarstedt, C. X. Andersson, and U. Smith. "Inflamed Adipose Tis-sue: A Culprit Underlying the Metabolic Syndrome and Atherosclerosis." *Arte-rioscler Thromb Vasc Biol* 27, no. 11 (2007): 2276–83.

Haarbo, J., U. Marslew, A. Gotfredsen, and C. Christiansen. "Postmenopausal Hormone Replacement Therapy Prevents Central Distribution of Body Fat after Menopause." *Metabolism* 40, no. 12 (1991): 1323–26.

Hahn, Frederick, Michael R. Eades, and Mary Dan Eades. *The Slow Burn Fitness Revolu-tion.* New York: Broadway Books, 2003.

Hamdy, O., S. Porramatikul, and E. Al-Ozairi. "Metabolic Obesity: The Paradox between Visceral and Subcutaneous Fat." *Curr Diabetes Rev* 2, no. 4 (2006): 367–73.

Hanley, A. J., and L. E. Wagenknecht. "Abdominal Adiposity and Diabetes Risk: The Im-portance of Precise Measures and Longitudinal Studies." *Diabetes* 57, no. 5 (2008): 1153–55.

Harris, R. B., and R. L. Leibel. "Location, Location, Location." *Cell Metab* 7, no. 5 (2008): 359–61.

Hollingsworth, K. G., M. Z. Abubacker, I. Joubert, M. E. Allison, and D. J. Lomas. "Low-Carbohydrate Diet Induced Reduction of Hepatic Lipid Content Observed with a Rapid Non-Invasive Mri Technique." *Br J Radiol* 79, no. 945 (2006): 712–15.

Jacobs, D., H. Blackburn, M. Higgins, D. Reed, H. Iso, G. McMillan, J. Neaton, J. Nel-son, J. Potter, B. Rifkind, and et al. "Report of the Conference on Low Blood Cho-lesterol: Mortality Associations." *Circulation* 86, no. 3 (1992): 1046–60.

Johnson, R. J., M. S. Segal, Y. Sautin, T. Nakagawa, D. I. Feig, D. H. Kang, M. S. Gersch, S. Benner, and L. G. Sanchez-Lozada. "Potential Role of Sugar (Fructose) in the Epi-demic of Hypertension, Obesity and the Metabolic Syndrome, Diabetes, Kidney Disease, and Cardiovascular Disease." *Am J Clin Nutr* 86, no. 4 (2007): 899–906.

Joiner, T. E., Jr., N. B. Schmidt, and D. Singh. "Waist-to-Hip Ratio and Body Dissatisfac-tion among College Women and Men: Moderating Role of Depressed Symptoms and Gender." *Int J Eat Disord* 16, no. 2 (1994): 199–203.

Jones, M. E., K. J. McInnes, W. C. Boon, and E. R. Simpson. "Estrogen and Adiposity—Utilizing Models of Aromatase Deficiency to Explore the Relationship." *J Steroid Biochem Mol Biol* 106, no. 1-5 (2007): 3–7.

Kim, S. P., M. Ellmerer, G. W. Van Citters, and R. N. Bergman. "Primacy of Hepatic Insulin Resistance in the Development of the Metabolic Syndrome Induced by an Isocaloric Moderate-Fat Diet in the Dog." *Diabetes* 52, no. 10 (2003): 2453–60.

Kortelainen, M. L., and T. Sarkioja. "Coronary Atherosclerosis Associated with Body Structure and Obesity in 599 Women Aged between 15 and 50 Years." *Int J Obes Relat Metab Disord* 23, no. 8 (1999): 838–44.

Kortelainen, M. L., and T. Sarkioja. "Extent and Composition of Coronary Lesions in Relation to Fat Distribution in Women Younger Than 50 Years of Age." *Arterioscler Thromb Vasc Biol* 19, no. 3 (1999): 695–99.

Kotronen, A., A. Seppala-Lindroos, R. Bergholm, and H. Yki-Jarvinen. "Tissue Specificity of Insulin Resistance in Humans: Fat in the Liver Rather Than Muscle Is Associated with Features of the Metabolic Syndrome." *Diabetologia* 51, no. 1 (2008): 130–38.

Kotronen, A., J. Westerbacka, R. Bergholm, K. H. Pietilainen, and H. Yki-Jarvinen. "Liver Fat in the Metabolic Syndrome." *J Clin Endocrinol Metab* 92, no. 9 (2007): 3490–97.

Kotronen, A., and H. Yki-Jarvinen. "Fatty Liver: A Novel Component of the Metabolic Syndrome." *Arterioscler Thromb Vasc Biol* 28, no. 1 (2008): 27–38.

Kullberg, J., C. von Below, L. Lonn, L. Lind, H. Ahlstrom, and L. Johansson. "Practical Approach for Estimation of Subcutaneous and Visceral Adipose Tissue." *Clin Physiol Funct Imaging* 27, no. 3 (2007): 148–53.

Kvist, H., B. Chowdhury, U. Grangard, U. Tylen, and L. Sjostrom. "Total and Visceral Adipose-Tissue Volumes Derived from Measurements with Computed Tomography in Adult Men and Women: Predictive Equations." *Am J Clin Nutr* 48, no. 6 (1988): 1351–61.

Lavine, J. E., and J. B. Schwimmer. "Nonalcoholic Fatty Liver Disease in the Pediatric Population." *Clin Liver Dis* 8, no. 3 (2004): 549–58, viii–ix.

Layman, D. K. "Protein Quantity and Quality at Levels above the Rda Improves Adult Weight Loss." *J Am Coll Nutr* 23, no. 6 Suppl (2004): 631S–36S.

———. "The Role of Leucine in Weight Loss Diets and Glucose Homeostasis." *J Nutr* 133, no. 1 (2003): 261S–67S.

Leao, L. M., M. P. Duarte, D. M. Silva, P. R. Bahia, C. M. Coeli, and M. L. de Farias. "Influence of Methyltestosterone Postmenopausal Therapy on Plasma Lipids, Inflammatory Factors, Glucose Metabolism and Visceral Fat: A Randomized Study." *Eur J Endocrinol* 154, no. 1 (2006): 131–39.

Lev-Ran, A. "Human Obesity: An Evolutionary Approach to Understanding Our Bulging Waistline." *Diabetes Metab Res Rev* 17, no. 5 (2001): 347–62.

Levine, J. A. "Nonexercise Activity Thermogenesis (Neat): Environment and Biology." *Am J Physiol Endocrinol Metab* 286, no. 5 (2004): E675–85.

———. "Nonexercise Activity Thermogenesis—Liberating the Life-Force." *J Intern Med* 262, no. 3 (2007): 273–87.

Levine, J. A., N. L. Eberhardt, and M. D. Jensen. "Role of Nonexercise Activity Thermogenesis in Resistance to Fat Gain in Humans." *Science* 283, no. 5399 (1999): 212–14.

Lobo, R. A. "Metabolic Syndrome after Menopause and the Role of Hormones." *Maturitas* 60, no. 1 (2008): 10–18.

Lovejoy, J. C., C. M. Champagne, L. de Jonge, H. Xie, and S. R. Smith. "Increased Visceral Fat and Decreased Energy Expenditure During the Menopausal Transition." *Int J Obes (Lond)* 32, no. 6 (2008): 949–58.

Maguire, L. S., S. M. O'Sullivan, K. Galvin, T. P. O'Connor, and N. M. O'Brien. "Fatty Acid Profile, Tocopherol, Squalene and Phytosterol Content of Walnuts, Almonds, Peanuts, Hazelnuts and the Macadamia Nut." *Int J Food Sci Nutr* 55, no. 3 (2004): 171–78.

Major, G. C., E. Doucet, P. Trayhurn, A. Astrup, and A. Tremblay. "Clinical Significance of Adaptive Thermogenesis." *Int J Obes (Lond)* 31, no. 2 (2007): 204–12.

Mastin, D. F., J. Bryson, and R. Corwyn. "Assessment of Sleep Hygiene Using the Sleep Hygiene Index." *J Behav Med* 29, no. 3 (2006): 223–27.

Mattsson, C., and T. Olsson. "Estrogens and Glucocorticoid Hormones in Adipose Tissue Metabolism." *Curr Med Chem* 14, no. 27 (2007): 2918–24.

McLean, J. A., S. I. Barr, and J. C. Prior. "Cognitive Dietary Restraint Is Associated with Higher Urinary Cortisol Excretion in Healthy Premenopausal Women." *Am J Clin Nutr* 73, no. 1 (2001): 7–12.

Mensink, R. P., J. Plat, and P. Schrauwen. "Diet and Nonalcoholic Fatty Liver Disease." *Curr Opin Lipidol* 19, no. 1 (2008): 25–29.

Mezey, E. "Dietary Fat and Alcoholic Liver Disease." *Hepatology* 28, no. 4 (1998): 901–905.

Miyashita, Y., N. Koide, M. Ohtsuka, H. Ozaki, Y. Itoh, T. Oyama, T. Uetake, K. Ariga, and K. Shirai. "Beneficial Effect of Low Carbohydrate in Low Calorie Diets on Visceral Fat Reduction in Type 2 Diabetic Patients with Obesity." *Diabetes Res Clin Pract* 65, no. 3 (2004): 235–41.

Munoz, J., A. Derstine, and B. A. Gower. "Fat Distribution and Insulin Sensitivity in Postmenopausal Women: Influence of Hormone Replacement." *Obes Res* 10, no. 6 (2002): 424–31.

Nanji, A. A., K. Jokelainen, G. L. Tipoe, A. Rahemtulla, and A. J. Dannenberg. "Dietary Saturated Fatty Acids Reverse Inflammatory and Fibrotic Changes in Rat Liver Despite Continued Ethanol Administration." *J Pharmacol Exp Ther* 299, no. 2 (2001): 638–44.

Nanji, A. A., S. M. Sadrzadeh, E. K. Yang, F. Fogt, M. Meydani, and A. J. Dannenberg. "Dietary Saturated Fatty Acids: A Novel Treatment for Alcoholic Liver Disease." *Gastroenterology* 109, no. 2 (1995): 547–54.

Nemetz, P. N., V. L. Roger, J. E. Ransom, K. R. Bailey, W. D. Edwards, and C. L. Leibson. "Recent Trends in the Prevalence of Coronary Disease: A Population-Based Autopsy Study of Nonnatural Deaths." *Arch Intern Med* 168, no. 3 (2008): 264–70.

Nielsen, J. V., and E. A. Joensson. "Low-Carbohydrate Diet in Type 2 Diabetes: Stable Improvement of Bodyweight and Glycemic Control During 44 Months Follow-Up." *Nutr Metab (Lond)* 5 (2008): 14.

Obici, S., and L. Rossetti. "Minireview: Nutrient Sensing and the Regulation of Insulin Action and Energy Balance." *Endocrinology* 144, no. 12 (2003): 5172–78.

Ogborne, A. C., and R. G. Smart. "Public Opinion on the Health Benefits of Moderate Drinking: Results from a Canadian National Population Health Survey." *Addiction* 96, no. 4 (2001): 641–49.

Ouyang, X., P. Cirillo, Y. Sautin, S. McCall, J. L. Bruchette, A. M. Diehl, R. J. Johnson, and M. F. Abdelmalek. "Fructose Consumption as a Risk Factor for Non-Alcoholic Fatty Liver Disease." *J Hepatol* 48, no. 6 (2008): 993–99.

Reiser, R. "Saturated Fat in the Diet and Serum Cholesterol Concentration: A Critical Examination of the Literature." *Am J Clin Nutr* 26, no. 5 (1973): 524–55.

Riechman, S. E., R. D. Andrews, D. A. Maclean, and S. Sheather. "Statins and Dietary and Serum Cholesterol Are Associated with Increased Lean Mass Following Resistance Training." *J Gerontol A Biol Sci Med Sci* 62, no. 10 (2007): 1164–71.

Rothacker, D. Q., B. A. Staniszewski, and P. K. Ellis. "Liquid Meal Replacement vs. Traditional Food: A Potential Model for Women Who Cannot Maintain Eating Habit Change." *J Am Diet Assoc* 101, no. 3 (2001): 345–47.

Saiki, A., Y. Miyashita, M. Wakabayashi, N. Kameda, and K. Shirai. "Reduction of Visceral Adiposity after Operation in a Subject with Insulinoma." *J Atheroscler Thromb* 11, no. 4 (2004): 209–14.

Sanchez-Mateos, S., C. Alonso-Gonzalez, A. Gonzalez, C. M. Martinez-Campa, M. D. Mediavilla, S. Cos, and E. J. Sanchez-Barcelo. "Melatonin and Estradiol Effects on Food Intake, Body Weight, and Leptin in Ovariectomized Rats." *Maturitas* 58, no. 1 (2007): 91–101.

Schmitz, K. H., P. J. Hannan, S. D. Stovitz, C. J. Bryan, M. Warren, and M. D. Jensen. "Strength Training and Adiposity in Premenopausal Women: Strong, Healthy, and Empowered Study." *Am J Clin Nutr* 86, no. 3 (2007): 566–72.

Schwimmer, J. B., R. Deutsch, T. Kahen, J. E. Lavine, C. Stanley, and C. Behling. "Prevalence of Fatty Liver in Children and Adolescents." *Pediatrics* 118, no. 4 (2006): 1388–93.

Schwimmer, J. B., R. Deutsch, J. B. Rauch, C. Behling, R. Newbury, and J. E. Lavine. "Obesity, Insulin Resistance, and Other Clinicopathological Correlates of Pediatric Nonalcoholic Fatty Liver Disease." *J Pediatr* 143, no. 4 (2003): 500–505.

Segal, M. S., E. Gollub, and R. J. Johnson. "Is the Fructose Index More Relevant with Regards to Cardiovascular Disease Than the Glycemic Index?" *Eur J Nutr* 46, no. 7 (2007): 406–17.

Sharma, S. V., J. A. Bush, A. J. Lorino, M. Knoblauch, D. Abuamer, G. Blog, and D. Bertman. "Diet and Cardiovascular Risk in University Marching Band, Dance Team and Cheer Squad Members: A Cross-Sectional Study." *J Int Soc Sports Nutr* 5 (2008): 9.

Sieminska, L., A. Cichon-Lenart, D. Kajdaniuk, B. Kos-Kudla, B. Marek, J. Lenart, and M. Nowak. "[Sex Hormones and Adipocytokines in Postmenopausal Women]." *Pol Merkur Lekarski* 20, no. 120 (2006): 727–30.

Singh, D. "Adaptive Significance of Female Physical Attractiveness: Role of Waist-to-Hip Ratio." *J Pers Soc Psychol* 65, no. 2 (1993): 293–307.

———. "Female Judgment of Male Attractiveness and Desirability for Relationships: Role of Waist-to-Hip Ratio and Financial Status." *J Pers Soc Psychol* 69, no. 6 (1995): 1089–101.

———. "Female Mate Value at a Glance: Relationship of Waist-to-Hip Ratio to Health, Fecundity and Attractiveness." *Neuro Endocrinol Lett* 23 Suppl 4 (2002): 81–91.

———. "Ideal Female Body Shape: Role of Body Weight and Waist-to-Hip Ratio." *Int J Eat Disord* 16, no. 3 (1994): 283–88.

———. "Waist-to-Hip Ratio and Judgment of Attractiveness and Healthiness of Female Figures by Male and Female Physicians." *Int J Obes Relat Metab Disord* 18, no. 11 (1994): 731–37.

Singh, D., P. Renn, and A. Singh. "Did the Perils of Abdominal Obesity Affect Depiction of Feminine Beauty in the Sixteenth to Eighteenth Century British Literature? Exploring the Health and Beauty Link." *Proc Biol Sci* 274, no. 1611 (2007): 891–94.

Smith, G. I., P. Atherton, D. T. Villareal, T. N. Frimel, D. Rankin, M. J. Rennie, and B. Mittendorfer. "Differences in Muscle Protein Synthesis and Anabolic Signaling in the Postabsorptive State and in Response to Food in 65-80 Year Old Men and Women." *PLoS ONE* 3, no. 3 (2008): e1875.

Solga, S., A. R. Alkhuraishe, J. M. Clark, M. Torbenson, A. Greenwald, A. M. Diehl, and T. Magnuson. "Dietary Composition and Nonalcoholic Fatty Liver Disease." *Dig Dis Sci* 49, no. 10 (2004): 1578–83.

Stefanovic-Racic, M., G. Perdomo, B. S. Mantell, I. J. Sipula, N. F. Brown, and R. M. O'Doherty. "A Moderate Increase in Carnitine Palmitoyltransferase 1a Activity Is Sufficient to Substantially Reduce Hepatic Triglyceride Levels." *Am J Physiol Endocrinol Metab* 294, no. 5 (2008): E969–77.

Stimson, R. H., A. M. Johnstone, N. Z. Homer, D. J. Wake, N. M. Morton, R. Andrew, G. E. Lobley, and B. R. Walker. "Dietary Macronutrient Content Alters Cortisol Metabolism Independently of Body Weight Changes in Obese Men." *J Clin Endocrinol Metab* 92, no. 11 (2007): 4480–84.

Symons, Donald. *The Evolution of Human Sexuality.* New York: Oxford University Press, 1981.

Szczepaniak, L. S., P. Nurenberg, D. Leonard, J. D. Browning, J. S. Reingold, S. Grundy, H. H. Hobbs, and R. L. Dobbins. "Magnetic Resonance Spectroscopy to Measure Hepatic Triglyceride Content: Prevalence of Hepatic Steatosis in the General Population." *Am J Physiol Endocrinol Metab* 288, no. 2 (2005): E462–68.

Tendler, D., S. Lin, W. S. Yancy, Jr., J. Mavropoulos, P. Sylvestre, D. C. Rockey, and E. C. Westman. "The Effect of a Low-Carbohydrate, Ketogenic Diet on Nonalcoholic Fatty Liver Disease: A Pilot Study." *Dig Dis Sci* 52, no. 2 (2007): 589–93.

Turcato, E., O. Bosello, V. Di Francesco, T. B. Harris, E. Zoico, L. Bissoli, E. Fracassi, and M. Zamboni. "Waist Circumference and Abdominal Sagittal Diameter as Surrogates of Body Fat Distribution in the Elderly: Their Relation with Cardiovascular Risk Factors." *Int J Obes Relat Metab Disord* 24, no. 8 (2000): 1005–10.

Voegtlin, Walter L. *The Stone Age Diet.* New York: Vantage Press, 1975.

Wei, Y., D. Wang, F. Topczewski, and M. J. Pagliassotti. "Fructose-Mediated Stress Signaling in the Liver: Implications for Hepatic Insulin Resistance." *J Nutr Biochem* 18, no. 1 (2007): 1–9.

Whitmer, R. A., D. R. Gustafson, E. Barrett-Connor, M. N. Haan, E. P. Gunderson, and K. Yaffe. "Central Obesity and Increased Risk of Dementia More Than Three Decades Later." *Neurology* 71, no. 14 (2008): 1057–64.

Yang, K., H. Guan, E. Arany, D. J. Hill, and X. Cao. "Neuropeptide Y Is Produced in Visceral Adipose Tissue and Promotes Proliferation of Adipocyte Precursor Cells Via the Y1 Receptor." *Faseb J* 22, no. 7 (2008): 2452–64.

Zamboni, M., E. Turcato, F. Armellini, H. S. Kahn, A. Zivelonghi, H. Santana, I. A. Bergamo-Andreis, and O. Bosello. "Sagittal Abdominal Diameter as a Practical Predictor of Visceral Fat." *Int J Obes Relat Metab Disord* 22, no. 7 (1998): 655–60.

SUBJECT INDEX

RECIPE INDEX